WHO NEEDS A GYM?

Using Social Media
For Weight Loss

ZHIVI WILLIAMS
Your Social Media Trainer

Leading by Example Publishing

ISBN: 978-0-692-65669-3

PRINTED IN THE UNITED STATES OF AMERICA

Worldwide, the obesity rate has doubled since 1980. There were 1.9 billion adults in 2014 that were overweight and these numbers are climbing every year. There's a clear need for a simple introduction to healthy living.

Who Needs a Gym, is written for those that don't know where to start on their healthy lifestyle journey. This book also included how to get free online healthy eating and weight loss support, meal suggestion, good and bad additives in foods, free workouts, mental strategies, detailed charts and resources along with recipes the reader can cook to help them live a healthy lifestyle.

In the pages of this book you will find the answers to the following questions:

- What foods should I eat to lose weight?
- What exercises should I do to lose weight?
- Should you pay for a gym membership, a personal trainer, start by walking, or find YouTube videos to do my workouts?
- How do I get rid of my belly?
- How often should I work out?
- What are some dishes I can cook?

"Zhivi is really leading by example in our group and on her side and of course, through her life! Thank you, Zhivi, for your beautiful BEING! The way you live has had an impact on my consistency in staying disciplined and not giving up. Your presence, compassion, sharing and honest feedback has given me so much. The journey goes on! Every day!" —Heike Fischer from Germany

"Zhivi is one of the most caring, inspirational women I know. She leads by example and constantly motivates others to be their best. Since she became a member of the TIFFANY ROTHE FITCLUB she has been a prominent example of what it means to be Fit, Fierce and Fabulous. I know she will be successful in teaching others to live healthier lives because she already is!" —Tiffany Rothe (Fitness Celebrity and CEO of the TIFFANY ROTHE FITCLUB)

Table of Contents

Thank You

First, I want to thank God for giving my husband the idea that I should write a book about my passion for living a healthy lifestyle. To my husband, Cleveland, thank you from the bottom of my heart. Thank you for seeing the possibilities inside of me and pull them out.

To my sister, Verletta, thank you for your support and for your honesty. You may not know it, but you are one of my role models.

I would also like to thank all my family members for supporting me and for giving me feedback when I needed it and especially when I didn't want it. In particular, thank you to my daughters, Yazimine Williams and Royal Clemonts.

To my brother, parents, best friend Samson, Lady, Sassy, Jael, Diamond, Coco and everyone that has helped on along my journey, supported me in all I have done and that I have learned a great deal from, thank you.

One scripture I have learned to stand on is Isaiah 55:11.

"It is better to strive to fulfill God's purpose for your life than to leave this earth with an overabundance of untapped potential and unattained blessings." Nikki R.

About the Author

Zhivi Williams is the founder of Leading by Example and Passion Driven, in Charlotte NC. Leading by Example's mission is to inspire change through health, wellness and fitness. Passion Driven's mission is to promote women's health and wellness through educational events.

On March 12, 2016, she hosted her first free Women's Health & Fitness Day in Charlotte, NC. The Women's Health & Fitness Day included vendors, interactive fitness classes and educational seminars highlighting the importance of living a healthy lifestyle from fitness and health experts.

She is a, motivational speaker, author, Health Coach, Personal Trainer, NASM certified Women's Fitness and Nutrition Specialist.

She was one of the featured stories on the Black Weight Loss Success website on August 2, 2014 (http://www.blackweightloss-success.com/more-than-weight-loss-zhivi-tranformed-her-body/#.U96XpWPQqM1).

She was also a contributing author for the book, The Driven Woman's Guide To A Fit Body, written by Ebonie Akinsete. She has also created the Fit & Over.... clothing line, which can be purchased on her website, www.leadingbyexample.us

We never know who is watching us and who will decide to change their lifestyle because of us. One of the best feelings in the world is when someone tells you, "Because of you, I have decided to eat healthy and lose some weight." You never know where this journey is going to take you, but as long as you continue on it through the ups and downs, good and bad times, you will accomplish what you have set out to do.

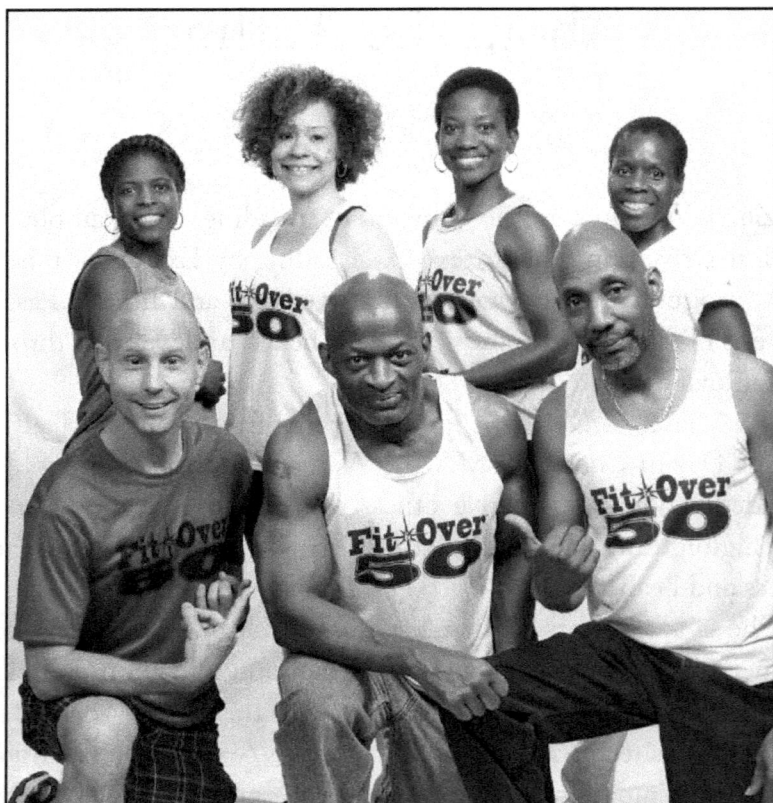

"And be not conformed to this world: but be you transformed by the renewing of your mind, that you may prove what is that good, and acceptable, and perfect, will of God. Romans 12:2

iv

Acknowledgements

To the members of my Facebook group page, Leading by Example, I would like to thank each and every person who has joined. I would also like to thank the following individuals for consistently posting encouraging comments to help us all on our healthy lifestyle journey: Michael, Cassive and Henry, thank you from the bottom of my heart.

When I started my healthy lifestyle journey, I just wanted to lose the fat around my stomach. As some readers may know, and some may not, you cannot "spot-lose" weight or fat. When you lose weight, you lose it from wherever your body is genetically predisposed to drop pounds. The first thing I did was look for a way to move. At the time I needed to work out at home, using exercise videos, even the grueling P90x plan. I did the entire workout, but I did not follow the eating plan and I wasn't getting the results I wanted. I worked out at home trying different programs for 20 months and none of them were giving me the results I wanted. I do want you to know that each of these programs came with a suggested meal plan to follow but I didn't think I needed to follow a meal plan. From my past experience with working out and eating whatever I wanted to, there was no need to follow a meal plan.

Because the workouts I was doing at home weren't working for me (I wasn't losing the weight and my stomach wasn't going down), I decided to find a program I could follow with a meal plan. After looking and searching, I found Tiffany Rothe Workouts. This was a God-send, straight from heaven. When I saw Tiffany's body I said,

"I can look like her." I was determined to follow her eating plan and workout schedule exactly as it was written. I had great success with the plan. I still do her workouts to this day, and I am now a Fitness Ambassador. I want to thank Tiffany and all of the Tiffany Rothe FitClub (TRFC) members for all of their support, motivation and honesty. Thank you, Tiffany, for being a great role model. You have shown me that all of us ladies have good days and bad days, including you, but when you have a bad day, the most important thing to do is to get back on track. I have learned so much from you and the TRFC members. Thank you for believing not only in yourself and in your vision for the TRFC, but for believing in us and encouraging us through our healthy lifestyle journey. You are truly a blessing to all women across the world. I know I am not going to be able to remember all of the wonderful members' names, but the ones I have seen act as an encouragement to others, while continuing to make great progress, who are Fit, Fierce and Fabulous: Robin M., Hemma, Daphna, Chris, Maria, Esme, Raphaëlle and all those that post daily. Not to just these members, but to all the members, keep up the great work.

Since joining the TRFC I have run a ½ marathon, become a NASM certified women's fitness specialist and nutrition specialist, gained more self-confidence, and even started my own business, Leading by Example (to help women live a healthy lifestyle through health, wellness and fitness) and a member of the Charlotte Mecklenburg County Women's Advisory Board. Through these, I have learned that I love to encourage and motivate people to take the best care of themselves that they can. I have also learned what it means to be happy with my body no matter how it looks. The TRFC has kept me going, from the phrase "Stay Focused" to the 3 C's: Constant, Consistent and Committed.

Sandi and the wonderful ladies of the Facebook page "Sisters in Fitness and Health (SIFH)" have also been a great support team for me. I joined this private Facebook page (at the time it was private) and have learned a great deal from Sandi Jackson. She is a very honest person who will ask you questions to make sure she understands where you are trying to go on your healthy lifestyle journey. Sandi, continue with the vision, you have a strong support system behind you. Because of the different groups under SIFH, you have made a difference in the lives of so many women. When you step out in faith, God will take care of you (I'm sure you know what I'm talking about). From this group of ladies, there are a number of them I would like to mention and to tell, "Keep doing what you are doing! Other people are watching you and they are making lifelong changes because of it." Keep up the great work, Izegbe, Regina, Hillery, Ethel, Xenia, Atiya, and all of the rest of the ladies I am unable to name.

Another support I am grateful for is the "African Americans Over 40, Fit & Fine" group. Not everyone in the group is African American, and anyone is welcome to join. There are people in this group who range from those just starting their journey to those who are bodybuilders. Not only are members supportive, but all members are allowed to express their opinions without conflict. Like any family, the people in the group have learned to agree to disagree. Thank you to Bre'e for starting this page. Those who have encouraged me to keep going and have given me great advice in the group are: Bre'e, Mijiza, Leonard, Keith, Sherwood, John, Otisa, Henri, Pamela, Aretha, Cassive, Johnny, Cawanda and Ayanna. Everyone in this group, keep working hard to meet your goals.

I would also like to thank Elyshia Brooks who has helped me to understand the importance of setting a date for my book to be published. Without her advice, I would have probably still be working on the book without a deadline.

I want to make sure I thank those who supplied their personal quotes on the pages on this book to keep you motivated on your journey. Special thank you to Brandi, Leonard, Aretha, Jacqueline,

Kenroy, Nicole, Michelle, Temple, Sherwood, Dennis, John, Sarah, Babette, Justina, Heike, Alex, Cawanda, Merna, Tanisha, Keith, Sandi, Vincent, Dr. Harriet, Johnny, Carlton, Ebonie, Charlies, Darius, Malgorzata, Karina, Cabrini, Dana, Tammie, Karen, Nikki, Rufus, Otisa, Paulina, Nick, Pamela, Ruby, See Jane Sweat, Dr. Verletta, CHarris, Cassive, Daphna, Eman, Kiran, Stephanie, Israel, Mishynn, Chris, Kimberly, Phillip, Casaline and Tabatha.

Some may wonder, why I have called so many people by name. I truly believe in giving honor where honor is do. Whether you are just starting out or have been on this healthy lifestyle journey for a while, keep up the great work. The one thing I have learned is that, you never know who is watching you and who will change their lifestyle because of you.

Foreword

One of the greatest gifts any student can give to her teacher is to apply what she has learned, not only to elevate her state of being, but also to breathe life into the dreams of others. Zhivi Williams is the perfect example of an exemplary student that has become an inspiration to everyone around her. She motivates, supports, and encourages people to be healthy and positive, and most importantly she leads by example. From the moment she joined "The TIFFANY ROTHE FITCLUB" I realized she was something special. She absorbed and implemented the principles of the plan and got amazing results, not only in her body, but in her state of mind. Zhivi was no ordinary student, she was exceptional, which is why she is now a great teacher. She personified my coaching mantra, which is to "Become the inspiration you seek". She used her positive experience to uplift everyone in the TRFC and all of those around her. There is not one active member that does not know her name, so it was no surprise when she became a fitness trainer herself. She is a natural motivator and a caring and informative coach.

When I read her book, I was impressed about her ability to take such important health and fitness related material and deliver it in small, easily digestible chunks of information. I highly recommend this book to anyone who wants to be healthy and fit. It will serve as a comprehensive "Go To" guide for questions about healthy eating, food additives, GMO's, workout options and more. So whether you are just starting with your fitness program or you are a fitness veteran in need of a motivational boost, reading this book will lift your spirit, educate your mind and help you to take the proper steps towards becoming the best you.

I endorse this reading for anyone who considers making the necessary changes for a healthy lifestyle.

Tiffany Rothe
CEO of the TIFFANY ROTHE FITCLUB

—◆—

*"When I look in the mirror I like what I see…
Working out gives me confidence to enjoy being me. I
don't have to look like anyone else. I just focus on being
my FIT, Fierce & Fabulous SELF!" Tiffany R.*

—◆—

The Mind Body Connection

Before you start reading this book, I want you to understand how stress and your mental health state can affect our healthy lifestyle journey.

Written by Dr. Verletta Saxon

I met with a man once who told me, "In every class I teach, I always tell people that you have to get your mind right before you can get your body right." I have held onto this truth to remember how important it is to make sure our minds and our bodies stay connected to achieve our physical, emotional and behavioral health goals. Distress, stress, and trauma can lead to a disruption in the way we think and behave, and in our moods. The CDC (Center for Disease Control) reports that about 50% of the population will have disruptions in the way they think, behave or mood at some point in their lives. These changes, including health concerns, can affect us socially, at work and in our personal lives. The health concerns associated with behavioral health are cardiovascular disease, diabetes, obesity, asthma, epilepsy, and cancer. In this chapter we will address the body's stress response, three common behavioral health concerns, and the benefits of exercise.

The Body's Stress Response

Emotional pain and physical pain are processed in the same region of the brain, and the body responds in the same way. The regions of the brain that respond to physical and emotional pain are the Amygdala and the hypothalamus. This area is so sensitive that it responds even to the thought of physical and emotional pain to produce the "fight, flight or freeze" response. During this response, the senses of smell, sight, hearing, taste and touch are all heightened and the body releases hormones to fend off the enemy. This response has been witnessed in mothers and fathers who have gained incredible strength to save their children and in soldiers who respond immediately to situations of danger to fight back.

When we as humans primarily lived outside among animals, the "fight, flight or freeze" response was essential to living. Humans were responsible for being on watch to protect themselves and their families from ravenous animals in the wild that might attack at any moment. It was important to know whether you should move, fight back, or run away from the animal or the situation. If a dangerous situation seemed imminent, the person's sense of smell, sight, hearing, taste and touch would become heightened and on the lookout for signs of attack. In addition to heightened senses, the body would physically get ready to respond. The heart would beat faster, breathing would speed up, hormones would be released, and muscles would tense. All of these physical responses evolved to help in life-threatening situations, preparing humans to fight or to flee the situation quickly. Once the threat of attack was over, they could go back to living the status quo, essentially living stress-free until the next threat of attack.

In today's society, the emotions that we experience activate the fight, flight or freeze response. But, unlike the response triggered by a physical situation, the emotional response is not limited to an hour, or a day; this response can go on for months, or years, and create an internal environment where our bodies feel like they are always under attack, resulting in chronic emotional pain, even physical illness. Some of the things that cause distress can be the loss of someone significant, stressful environments, sexual orientation, money, work, traffic, accidents, bullying, and/or rejection from society, peers, and loved ones. When we experience emotional or physical danger, the "fight, flight or freeze" response can result in the following:

Fight

The body gets ready to fight whatever danger is present.

Flight

The body prepares to leave a threatening situation.

Freeze

Response is minimal; individuals are stuck in a way that does not allow them to move from the situation.

Repeated activation of the stress response, research has found, can cause long-term effects that affect the body and mind. Prolonged stress has been associated with health conditions such as high blood pressure, cancer, heart attacks, addictions, sleep and eating disorders, obesity, anxiety and depression.

———◦———

"From the stem to the gym." Carlton S. (I was a crack cocaine smoker and the pipe we used was called a stem. After I got clean and in shape some of my former dealers were really proud of me, actually amazingly, a few would say man I'm so happy for you bro. Some of them were struggling to, so I would see them and I would say "from the stem to the gym.").

———◦———

Post-Traumatic Stress Disorder

Post-Traumatic Stress Disorder is thought to be a condition where the "fight, flight or freeze" response is always turned on. The person experiencing this kind of emotional trauma is constantly on watch for an attack. The intensity of the emotion they experience can be very high, which makes the response very intense. The original event that brings on this type of stress is typically one that is traumatizing for that person. For example, a car accident could traumatize a person to the point that they are no longer able to ride in a vehicle or to sit in the passenger seat without having a physical reaction every time the vehicle stops. I have been in several major car accidents over time, including one accident where a tire blew out on a busy highway and our vehicle spun around in circles. However, while I remember the accident, I was not traumatized by it. I once rode in a vehicle with a friend who had had an accident where she was not injured, but nevertheless the event was traumatizing for her. She is fully capable of driving, but when she is a passenger in a vehicle, her heart rate immediately goes up, her palms become sweaty, and every time the vehicle stops, she grasps her seat and moves as if to make the vehicle stop. She is so scared that she will have another car accident that she is constantly preparing for that accident in her mind. We see these same reactions in individuals who have grown up in environments where they needed to be prepared to fend off what they would consider an enemy, like violent family members, as well as in soldiers. The important thing to remember is that what traumatizes one person may not traumatize another.

Anxiety

Anxiety is a feeling of inner turmoil or unrest about a future event. It is often associated with worry and an impending sense of doom about what might happen in the future. Take the following examples of anxiety: a neighbor or a friend who is concerned about a child's leaving for college, about whether the child is prepared to take on this new challenge in life, or another who is concerned about how their bills will get paid, or it could be your turn to give a speech in front of thousands of people. Just that thought alone sends most people into a state of anxiety! In these situations, a person is concentrating on future events that might happen instead of what is occurring at the moment. Anxiety can be an underlying condition of some health problems, such as heart or lung conditions. Constant worry and anxiety can lead to problems concentrating, fatigue and can tense all muscle groups but some of the typical muscles are your shoulders and neck.

Depression

Countless individuals suffer from depression on a daily basis. Depression can be associated with underlying medical conditions, substance abuse, death or the loss of something or someone important, major life events, a serious illness, abuse, a family history. The CDC estimates that 1 in 10 adults has depression in America. Typical signs of depression are low self-esteem, a loss of interest in activities that were once enjoyable or desirable, feelings of worthlessness, a loss of appetite, problems concentrating and remembering. When individuals are depressed they are often focused only on what has happened in the past.

Anxiety, depression and PTSD are conditions that can be experienced by anyone and that affect our daily lives. Even when working out and eating well to combat them, these conditions affect our motivation and our will to go on. In the following sections I discuss some ways to deal with these conditions.

How Exercise Can Help

Our bodies and brains are interconnected and work together for optimal mental and physical health. What we think determines how we react; our mind helps us solve problems and remember solutions. Physical activity influences the brain by relieving stress. The process of physical exercise involves techniques similar to meditation, such as deep breathing, which relieves muscle tension and improves mental focus to produce a calming effect. Hormones are also released that produce pleasurable sensations.

Movement and exercise can also help us learn to stay in the moment instead of concentrating on past, or future, events. It can also help us find new ways to solve problems, which can result in inner peace, rejuvenation, and transformation of mental state.

Exercise releases endorphins like dopamine that produce feelings of happiness, excitement and satisfaction. These endorphins respond to stress, pain and fear by blocking pain and controlling emotional responses. When these endorphins work correctly, they send signals to our bodies to discontinue the actions causing pain, or they produce chemicals to let us know an activity is something pleasurable and enjoyable. Exercise creates a sense of well-being and, as we exercise, chemicals are produced in the body that are pleasurable. Studies have found that 30 minutes of exercise 3 or more times a week has been found to reduce or eliminate depression and anxiety symptoms, to improve one's self image or self-worth, and to increase self-esteem. To get the greatest feeling of happiness or excitement, exercise should be intense, or should feature a period(s) of increased exertion.

Relaxation Techniques

Deep breathing, peaceful words and situations, visualization, prayer, yoga, and other relaxation techniques have been proven to be effective at fighting off the stress response and reducing blood pressure. While this may not be a cure, it has been proven to reduce those physical symptoms related to stress.

Getting Additional Help

Similar to seeking out help for physical health needs, getting help for behavioral health needs can guide you to successfully manage stress, distress and help you achieve your goals. If we treat our physical and our behavioral health together, this leads to better outcomes and helps to achieve our goals. Individuals who can help with behavioral health concerns include counselors, psychiatrists, social workers, substance abuse counselors, peer support specialists, psychologists, sociologists and primary care physicians. They can help address behavioral health issues that come up in your life and also help you develop coping skills and solutions to emotional issues. If you are experiencing an emotional crisis, such that you are not able to control your emotions or you cannot express your emotions, please find the nearest Behavioral Health Crisis Center or a local Emergency Center for immediate services. Assistance is also available by phone or online at the National Suicide Prevention Lifeline.

"Opportunities for growth disguise themselves as disappointment, emotional pain, and fear. Face each disappointment, pain, and fear with the confidence that you can win and you will grow." Dr. Verletta S.

How Support Can Help

Support Groups

Support groups can be found at your local gym or on social media. Support groups can focus on different topics and are often as ways to support a person's daily life. Support groups may be called running groups, healthy eating groups, powerlifting clubs, group fitness, and weight loss groups just to name a few. People often make connections in these groups that help them maintain a healthy lifestyle, stay motivated, be held accountable, and set personal goals.

Motivation

Let's face it, most people start out strong but do not always finish strong. We set goals of losing 10, 20, 30, or more pounds but everyday life gets in the way of those goals. Sometimes we worked longer hours than we thought we would, the kids have soccer practice, or you are exhausted and feel like you cannot do one more thing by the end of the day. Working out in supportive groups can help you set goals and achieve those goals. As humans we are geared toward group activities. Those groups may be large 100,000 people or as small as one other person, but we are comfortable in group settings. In a group, the leader sets the pace and the rest of the group put their energy toward meeting the request of the leader, this challenge keeps them motivated and energized to meet their goals.

Group Challenges

When setting goals in a group, one of the goals is to challenge your body to do more than you were previously able to accomplish. To run longer, to lift more weight, to increase the pace, or to do a new exercise so that your body does not plateau. We push ourselves so that we can improve and reach our fitness goals. Meeting the challenge of the change in exercise gives us a sense of accomplishment and when done in a group can be motivation for ourselves and others to continue working out until we are able to reach the next challenge and complete the program.

Accountability

When working out in groups we are held accountable from the inside out and from the outside in. When we are holding ourselves accountable we are working from the inside out. We set goals for ourselves and dream of how we will look when we have reached our goals. While this is an effective method of holding ourselves accountable, sometimes we become overwhelmed with life and need someone else to encourage us to reach our fitness goals. When working in groups, we set our own internal goals, but the group helps to keep us accountable to attending the group, simply by expecting us to show up. If someone in the group has not been seen in a while someone is reaching out to them in order to encourage them or to ensure that nothing is wrong.

Chapter 1
You Can't Do It Alone

So you want to get healthy. That's great! I'm here to help. And if there's one thing I've learned about getting healthy, it is that you need help to get there in the first place and to stay that way consistently. I have compiled this book to help those looking to increase their fitness level, eat a bit healthier, lose weight, feel better and to make a lifestyle change. I believe that the best way to do this is through connecting to others, as well as connecting to yourself.

We are all looking for someone to motivate us, hold us accountable, tell us to keep going when we don't want to and for people not to judge us as we tackle this health, wellness and fitness journey (what I like to call, living a healthy lifestyle). What better way to do this than through connecting with online communities through social media.

'If it does not work say "OH well" it's better then
never trying and saying "What if"' Cabrini S.

Social media a great way to connect with people that are like-minded. People who have been where you are, can encourage and motivate you to reach your goals. The best part of connecting with people through online communities is, IT'S FREE. Who doesn't like getting something for free? You will get free advice, encouragement, motivation, recipes, suggested workouts, and a community of people who will not judge you if you fall down.

This healthy lifestyle journey is a process and if you can connect with like-minded people on your journey it will make the journey a little easier. Being a part of an online community can also help you to find the process that works for you. What one person might do to get to where they are on their journey may not be the same process that works for you. But being a part of a community gives you the opportunity to try different things that may or may not work. You will find a process that works for you and that process will help you to reach your goals.

Although you may walk this journey alone (you have to put in the work, no one can put it in for you) you don't have to do it alone. You will need the encouragement of others, people you can look to for advice, people to pull you up when you have fallen down and motivation from people who tell you, "If I can do it, you can also" The one thing I love seeing in an online fitness and health community are before and after pictures. This shows everyone, if they can do it, so can the next person.

———————

'When someone or something is trying to get in the way of your workout, keep one thing in mind: "Nobody messes with my workout. BOOYAH!" You're the boss of you.'
Daphna S.

———————

Don't you want people to encourage you and tell you that you are doing a great job? Everyone does and you will get this from the online community. But you have to be willing to share your pictures

and make a collage of your progress. I know this may be embarrass-
ing at first, but, you have to love yourself where you are so that as you
go through the process, others will see how much you love yourself.
Never be embarrassed at where you start because everyone has a
starting point. Sometimes the best way to get that encouragement
is to post a start pictures (which also helps with accountability) or
a picture after you workout to get those encouraging words that we
all love to hear.

Everyone that decides to live a healthy lifestyle has to go through
a process and a journey. First, I'd like to share my own journey as well
as those of others, to remind you that you are not the first person to
ever start out on one of these journeys. Never judge anyone's starting point because we all start out having to change what we eat and
exercise and that is not always easy.

Chapter 2
Weight Loss Journey

My Personal Journey

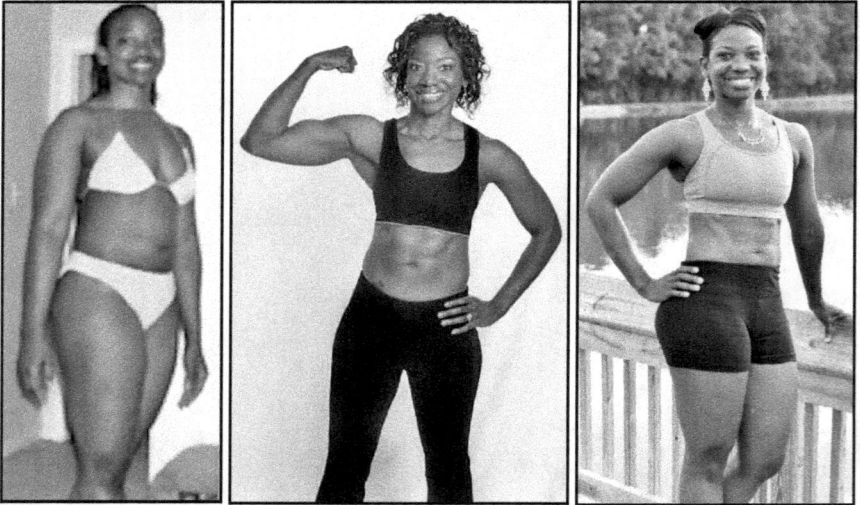

Let's start with me: I started my journey in the fourth grade. My doctor told my mom that my motor skills weren't developed, which was why I had a hard time remembering what I was taught in school, and that exercising would help me.

In fourth grade I was labeled with a learning disability and went into special education classes that were taught at a slower pace. I stayed in special education until my junior year in high school, when I was able to switch to regular classes with the other students.

"If you wish for something good, it's already yours but you have to reach for it." Malgorzata Ch.

In fourth grade I played softball, which I loved. From 4th grade to 6th grade I swam. However, during junior high, at that time, 7th and 8th grade, I didn't play a sport. And in those years, my grades suffered. Although my motor skills had started to develop in elementary school, I still needed to exercise to continue to develop my motor skills.

In high school I was on the swimming and gymnastics teams as well. My sophomore through senior years, I focused only on the gymnastics team and practiced year round. At this time I also started lifting weights. Participating in these activities had a huge beneficial effect. The more active I was, the better my grades were. So much so that, by the time I was a junior, I could make the change from special education classes to regular classes, because my memory, and grades, had improved so much.

When I first attended college, I thought I would not need to exercise anymore. I continued lifting weights sporadically, but the lack of exercise really affected my grades. For a while I didn't notice, but once I made the connection, I decided it was time to start working out. I started going to the weight room and when I did, my grades improved.

———◉———

"...inspire til you expire..." Alex K.

———◉———

After graduating from college, in December of 1996, I consistently worked out until 2005. During this time period, I wasn't eating healthfully because I was active and not gaining weight. In 2005, I became pregnant. After the delivery of my son, it was hard to get back on track. Eventually, though, I did lose the weight I had gained, even though I was still not consistently working out and wasn't eating healthfully.

Between 2005 and 2011, I worked out but not on a consistent basis. I would do well at first. I would get up some mornings, go to the gym, exercise for at least an hour and feel great. But after some time, laziness would set in and I would stop working out in the mornings. I would continue this cycle over the next 6 years.

In 2011, I became pregnant again. I was older (37), and my body wasn't dropping the weight as easily as it had done in the past. I started my pregnancy at 148 pounds. When I delivered my son, I weighed 173 pounds. Eventually, I got back down to 150 pounds, but I wasn't happy with the way my body looked, specifically my stomach. I started again, doing several different exercise videos at home, but I was not consistent and I had not changed my eating habits.

———◉———

"Adjust your eating habits and workout routines in accordance with your injuries and or illnesses. Don't just give up totally. If you can't work lower body, work upper body. If you can't run, walk. Just keep moving and continue to eat clean." Keith B.

———◉———

One way I was sabotaging myself was that I would eat at fast food restaurants at least 5-6 times a week. When I was out, going to work, going home, or running around, when I got hungry I would stop and get a little cheap and quick snack. I hadn't yet realized how much it was affecting my body and hindering my weight loss.

Another way was how I was working out off and on. I thought if I worked out a little bit—like I did in my 20s—I could lose the weight. I soon found out, that wasn't true. I wasn't going to lose the weight from working out alone.

In December of 2012, I decided to take losing weight, and my health, seriously. I shared my plan with certain people and they told me I didn't need to lose weight. That was kind of them to say, but I was on a journey to make my stomach look like it did when I was 27 years old.

One day I found Tiffany Rothe workouts. She offered exactly what I was looking for, and she looked the way I wanted to look. When I saw her, I said, "If she can look like that, so can I." I joined her Tiffany Rothe FitClub (TRFC). After joining the TRFC, I shared a photograph of myself at 27 with Tiffany Rothe and told her, "This is what I want my stomach to look like." She told me that it would look *better* than that picture. I believed her and started out following the workouts and eating plan to a tee.

"Always believe in yourself, even when others can't"
Tabatha "Gigi" W.

I was determined to put in the time and commitment to get the results I wanted. I started taking pictures of myself every four weeks so I could see my progress. This was the first time in my life that

I had worn a bikini (and let other people see me in one). I trusted the ladies in the TRFC, so I posted the pictures and shared them with other members. I would wear the same bikini for months. One day, Tiffany and one of the other ladies of the TRFC told me it was time for a new bikini because the one I had been taking pictures in was too big. It's funny how when we lose weight, we continue to wear the clothes we started out in, not realizing they are too big. Some of us don't realize they are too big until they fall down (has that ever happened to you?). Over the next few months I went from 149 to my lost weight of 127 pounds. During this process my confidence level rose and in the summer of 2013, for the first time, ever, in my life I decided to wear a bikini in public. The experience was a little awkward, but I did it and I was proud of myself for doing it because I no longer had a complex about how my body looked.

My journey has been filled with ups and down. My husband, coworkers, and friends all told me at different times that I was losing too much weight and that I should stop. I kept going because I am the one that has to live with this body, and I wanted it to look a certain way. I kept working out and following the food plan that was given to me, and no matter what anyone said I was going to keep going until I thought I was too small. Once I weighed 127 lbs. (57.60 kilos), which was too small even for me, I began the process of gaining weight back, but not by eating unhealthy foods, but through weight lifting. My plan now is to build muscle instead of focusing on weight loss. I don't mind going up in weight as long as it is not from fat. Not only do I track my weight, but more importantly, I track my body fat percentage. I am currently at 20.2 % body fat.

"Don't follow your dreams, because dreams happen while you sleep. Follow your passions, because your passion is the reason you were created!" Sarah H.

I have accomplished much more than I ever thought I would on this healthy lifestyle journey. Although it started out about transforming my stomach, my journey ended up with my earning certificates as both a women's fitness specialist and a fitness nutrition specialist. I also learned that I love to motivate other individuals on their healthy lifestyle journey. At some points, we all need someone to motivate and encourage us to keep going. If you are looking for someone to hold you accountable and motivate you, visit my website at www.leadingbyexample.us and sign up for a 30 minute free coaching session. I also ran my first half marathon in November 2013. This is something I never thought I would do, nor had I ever planned on running so far, but I decided to challenge myself. I ran the half marathon in 2:18 with minimal training. I could have done much better if I trained for the race. I have also done personal training and radio interviews, neither of which would have been possible without my experience in fitness.

Through all this, I've learned the importance of living this lifestyle in front of others. We never know who is watching us and who will decide to change their eating and exercise behaviors because of us. One of the best feelings in the world is when someone tells you, "Because of you, I have decided to eat well and lose some weight." You never know where this journey is going to take you, but as long as you continue on it through the ups and downs, the good and bad times, you will accomplish what you have set out to do. Remember, living a healthy lifestyle is something you do for the rest of your life;

it is not a diet. You don't "complete it" once you reach your goals. Once you achieve your goal weight, you have to continue to do what you are doing to maintain your goal weight. If you don't, the weight will begin to creep back on and usually you gain more than what you started with.

———◦◦———

"Do what your personal trainer/coach tells u to do" John W.

———◦◦———

Just to let you know, I have my share of ups and downs, and there are always things I can do better, especially drinking more water. Drinking a lot of water is a struggle for me. I have given into temptation at times, by drinking soda, but I don't let that keep me down. I get up and get back on the plan. There are days I have to force myself to workout, but I get up and get it done. I always feel better afterwards. If you have fallen down, it is time to get back up and start again. I promise you will feel better. To start living a healthy lifestyle, through healthy eating and exercise, follow me on social media Facebook: Zhivi Williams, Twitter: LBX Fitness, Instagram: LBX Fitness, and Pinterest: LBX Fitness. Please visit my website for speaker engagments and health coachign services, www.leadingbyexample.us. Please visit our website to learn more about our speaking services.

Keith's Personal Journey

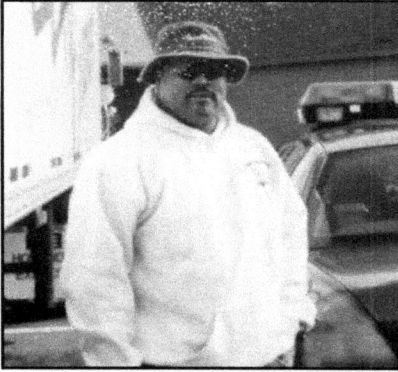

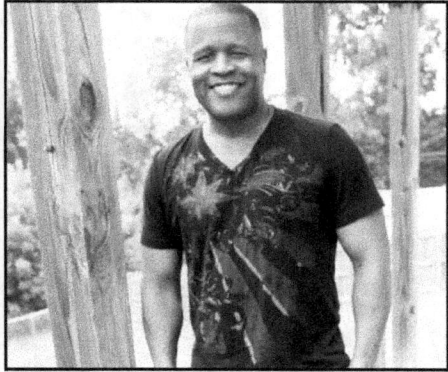

In 2003 I was diagnosed with high blood pressure and diabetes after experiencing dizzy spells. I started to eat clean and work out. I did only the treadmill for a few years, then I added weight lifting. I was on high blood pressure and diabetes medication until 2011/2012, when I decided to become vegetarian, while continuing my workouts. My doctor took me off the high blood pressure and diabetes medications because I took the initiative to start eating healthfully and working out. In 2014, I became a Vegan and I'm still working out and eating clean.

———◆———

"As you begin your fitness journey, you are ultimately responsible for achieving the desired fitness and health results. Your friends and family may fall off the bandwagon so you need to become your own motivator and personal trainer from within to continue for a lifetime." Keith B.

———◆———

Meriem's Personal Journey

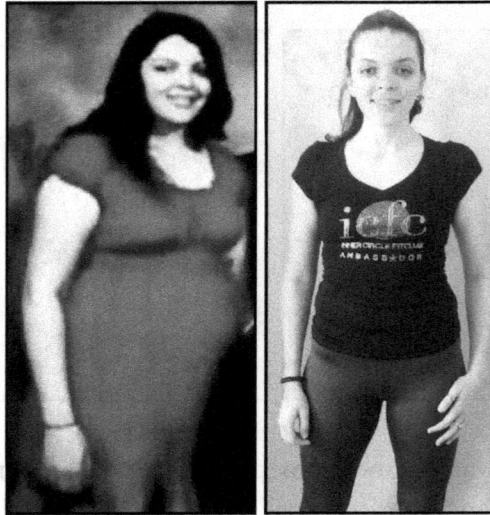

"Don't let those too afraid to dream, crush yours."
See Jane Sweat

Growing up, I have always been a little on the chubby side. I managed to get that under control in my teenage years by taking up running and cycling to school together with a healthy diet; I did quite well and felt great then! But things started to spiral out of control when I went to university and started living alone. Little by little old bad habits and new, even worse, ones started creeping up and settling in, and before I knew it pizza and other processed ready meals became my norm. At some point I decided to enroll in a 6 weeks on-campus weight management program. I did pretty well but being in a "diet" mindset I did not keep it up after those 6 weeks, even though it was an easy-to-follow program that was based on healthy eating and regular exercise. Going back to my old habits, I gained all the weight I lost and some more! My worst was sometime around 2010 when I hit 106kg (234 lbs). Leading up to that, I had been dieting on and off and starting exercise programs that I did not finish. My real breakthrough came after a medical check-up where I was diagnosed as being pre-diabetic with signs of high blood pressure to top it off. That terrified me, especially with my family history with those diseases! My doctor suggested putting me on medication, but to me that was out of the question! I knew that was enough and that I had to take drastic measures and make permanent lifestyle changes. I started slow, first by cutting out junk food and walking everyday, then I gradually increased the intensity of my workouts with regular jogs as I lost weight. The best was when I came across one of Tiffany Rothe's free workouts on YouTube; I quickly became addicted and got great results! After that I decided to join her full program with integrated eating and workout plans and that's when magic happened! Nearly three years down the line, I am still with her and most importantly I am still leading a healthy lifestyle! I am now in the best shape of my life both physically and mentally, I really believe that I gained a lot more than all the weight I lost and in many aspects of my life! My blood pressure is now comparable to an athlete's and I am now definitely in the clear with regards to diabetes risks. This is definitely the best and the most precious gift I have ever given to myself! The most important thing for me was to realize that this is not just about looking good or about the number on the scale. Having those things as my sole motivators was probably the reason why I never stuck to a healthy longterm weight loss program. The key for me was to know that, to get to a position where I am able to make the right choices for a better and healthier me, I had to start by finding true love and respect for myself and my body. I would have never broken the crash diet cycle otherwise, and I would still be unhealthy and unhappy. This is not about dieting or about quick fixes. This is for life, and I would not have it any other way!

Rae's Personal Journey

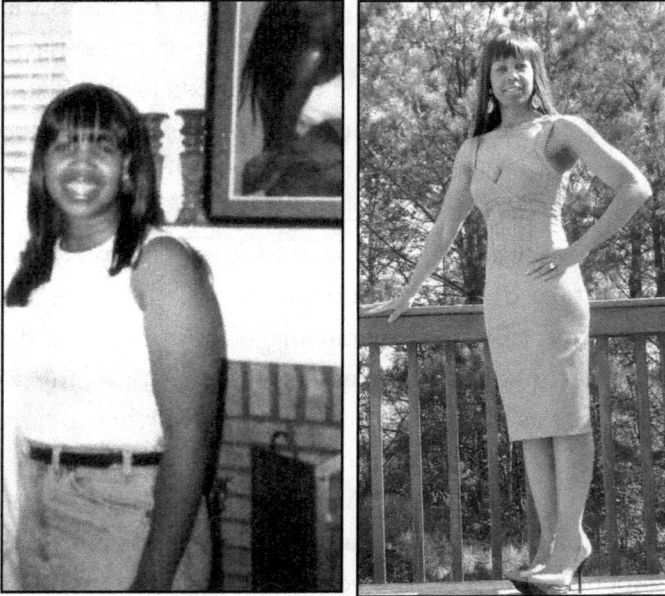

I began my weight loss journey in 2005. After maintaining a 160-pound body for over 10 years, I quickly ballooned to 225-pounds after transitioning from corporate America to self-employment. It took me almost three years to shed the weight and reach my weight loss goal of 135 pounds. I took the slow and steady road, which resulted in minimal hanging skin.

My weight gain did not become evident to me until I attempted to wear an outfit that "I thought" highlighted my body. In fact, it did not fit. I decided to make a change.

—◦—

"Don't prove them wrong.
Prove your negative thoughts wrong."
Zhivi W.

—◦—

Although the media shunned Kevin Trudeau (the television personality), his message resonated in my psyche, caught my attention and was instrumental in changing my life. I transitioned from conventional to organic food. At the time, I was a whopping 225 pounds. I discarded conventional, refined-sugar, MSG-contained foods and replaced them with organic, natural, unprocessed foods. After changing the foods housed in my cupboard, the internet became my primary source of information. I researched food toxins, detoxification, portions control, food tracking, cardio and strength training. I even joined websites that contain weight-conscious individuals. Joining these websites enabled me to track my progress, communicate with those in process of losing weight and admire those who reached their weight loss goals. Interacting via internet allowed me to document my new lifestyle and become accountable for my good and challenging nutritional choices.

———◁◉▷———

"Each unique pearl represents an untold
story of your valor." Pamela R.

———◁◉▷———

In the beginning of 2012, I opened a new business and in 2013, I enrolled in a doctoral program. The extra responsibilities compromised my workouts. My two-hour daily workouts were substituted with reading, writing and internet research. At the beginning of 2014, I noticed a twelve-pound weight gain. Although I adhere to a relatively clean diet, my body took a new turn without regular exercise. My size 2 and 4 dresses are snug and I have noticed some extra cushion around my midsection. In the summer of 2014, I took time from school to focus on my businesses, but also to revamp my schedule to allow my businesses, doctoral studies *and* fitness.

As of September 2, 2014, classes have resumed, but I will continue my fitness journey as I am reminded that a clean diet alone does not equate to a fit body. Only the combination of effective cardiovascular training and strength training produces the result of a fit body.

————◎————

"Fighting for yourself proves you're worth fighting for."
Sarah H."

————◎————

Pushkal's Personal Journey

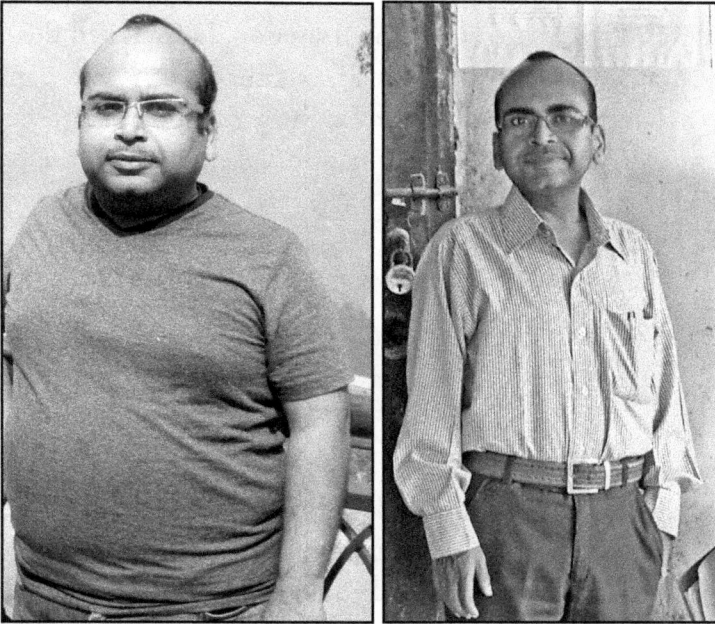

I have been obese since childhood. People, when they saw me, would start laughing. I felt embarrassment when going in public. Having a fit body has been my dream, flat abs have always been distant dream that never came true for me. I tried everything from dieting, workouts, joining the gym, yoga, to peels. Then, a year ago, I saw videos of Tiffany Rothe workouts. After trying her booty shaking workout, I joined her Tiffany Roth FitClub following. I started following the workouts and diet plan. Within 6 months, my weight reduced from 78 (172 lbs) to 46 kg (102 lbs) and my waistline from 38 inch to 30 inch. I even got flat abs. However, there were lot of ups and downs in achieving this goal. I love to eat fried foods and ice cream. As a legal professional in a prestigious institution, I have to attend many meetings where snacks and salty foods are served. I was determined not to eat them, and after time, people began to understand that I will not eat unhealthy foods. Gradually they stopped trying to serve those foods to me. But sometimes I fell into the temptation of eating ice cream. Later on, I developed the mindset that I am not depriving myself, but that I choose a conscious path to stay fit. Now I check my weight regularly and also perform a cleanse every month. I am very happy and now I have the body of my dreams.

———◉———

"Food is fuel, no more no less." Temple T

———◉———

Further to my story, I want to share with you that sometimes in the past people avoided me because of my bad physique. In my family, I was often ignored. But after my transformation everyone admires the change in my body. People also appreciate my determination to take in only healthy food.

Heike's Personal Journey

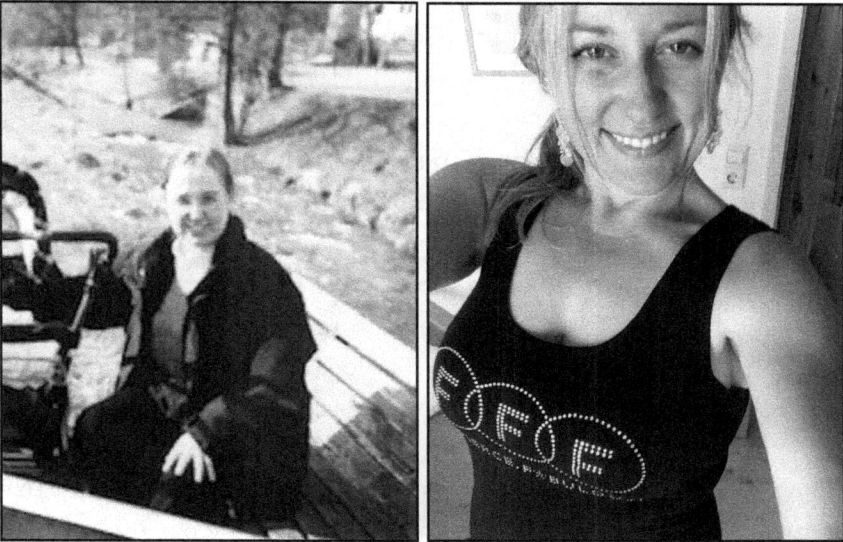

"I believe in giving 100% in the areas of improvement you want 100% in. Not 80% here, 30% there. Go full throttle baby!" CHarris ~ CHEKnows Wellness, Fitness & Lifestyle Expert

---

After the birth of my son I put on weight and, although I did some aerobics twice a week, I still didn't lose the weight. The years between 2001 and 2006, I was the heaviest. I am 1.62 m (5'3") and weighed almost 70 kilos (154 lbs) in that summer. I admit that my whole life started to change in the next 2 years. I sank deeper into "The Work of Byron Katie", a process to question stressful beliefs. In pursuing that, I decided to care for my body, too. I did a course in healthy nutrition and started jogging. Then it was very bad weather and I was looking for some workouts on YouTube. I found Tiffany Rothe and loved her workouts because I saw results, and they were fun. I lost some weight and felt better. I completed three 5k races and one 10k. Then I started to go to dance classes after a musical further education workshop. Tiffany's words have motivated me to work out almost every day and to trust myself. I have noticed that I have gained more and more confidence. All of a sudden I saw on Tiffany's video that people can subscribe to her program and I did it. I love and hate and love the journey! I am now in and plan to stay in.

It is 2014 now and I have lost 10 kilos (22 lbs) slowly and steadily. I feel much younger than 43 and my eating habits have changed to a healthy and delicious life style. My results are not only visible in the way I look but my doctor says that I have athletic data and that I am very healthy! My self-esteem and consistency has improved in all areas of my life! So grateful for the lesson!

———◆———

"If there was one word or phrase to live by, it is love. Love yourself, love your life, and it will be easy to love others." Rufus M.

———◆———

Chapter 3
The First Step to Being Successful on Your Journey

After having read a bunch of success stories, you are probably ready to get going on your own journey. You may have noticed how many of these people mentioned their mindset as key to unlocking their potential and best selves.

Most fitness books begin by talking about healthy food, or workouts. Those are very important parts of weight loss or a healthy lifestyle (and we will discuss those later on), but first let's begin by talking about the most important (and most-overlooked) aspect affecting weight loss and health: Your mind. How you think about yourself, and your journey, will determine your success.

———◈———

"If this is Hard for me I Know It's Hard For You" John W.

———◈———

Change the Way You Think

"The first place we lose the battle is in our own thinking. If you think it's permanent then it's permanent. If you think you've reached your limits then you have. If you think you'll never get well then you won't. You have to change your thinking. You need to see everything that's holding you back, every obstacle, every limitation as only temporary." —Joel Osteen

One of the hardest things you will face on this healthy lifestyle journey is changing the way you think. No one is exempt from the negative thoughts about eating unhealthy food—"I wish this was a cheeseburger"—or not wanting to work out ("I'd rather watch TV"). How you handle these thoughts will be the difference between success and giving up.

When you start thinking things like "It's too early," "I can't get up," "I will start tomorrow," "This isn't working," "It is too hard," this is when you have to start telling yourself the opposite. When you think, "It is too early," tell yourself, "Well, if I get up now and work out, I can take a nap later."

What I have found is that, when people wait to work out later in the day, if they usually work out in the morning, they don't end up working out later because they get too tired or too busy by the end of the day. Sometimes you have to just force yourself to get up. I have had to do this on many days—but once I am up and moving around, I am ready to work out.

"If you want change, you have to make change"
And don't sit around singing the I should of, could of,
would of song." Tammie R.

Motivating yourself to push harder also requires a change in your thinking. Having a personal trainer is great, because he or she is going to push you to wake up, to show up, and to do one more rep, but if you are in the gym by yourself, you are going to have to push on your own, when you want to give up.

I work out alone and there are times where I have created a routine for myself and I get to a certain point where I say, "I am tired and I really don't have to do this last set." Then I say, "You made this routine up and you said you were going to do it, so let's get it done." I push out the last set or routine. Then it's done.

I will also ask someone to spot me in the gym if I need the spot. When you work out alone, it is difficult to push that last set out once you start to struggle. I look around the gym to see if I can tell if someone knows what they are doing before I ask someone to spot me. Once I find someone, I just walk up and ask. Don't be scared to ask for help because it will help with thinking "I can't do any more."

Let's say, while taking a class, you are getting tired and feel like you can't go on. Don't give up! Slow down, take a small break then jump back in. When I first started doing Tiffany Rothe Workouts, there were some videos where I just had to stop because my muscles were burning or because I was tired. I would stop for maybe 30 seconds to a minute, then I would get back into the work out. I would not stop the video, I would let it play and start where ever she was. I kept doing this until I was strong enough to do the full video workout without stopping.

———————

"Imagine each step as a glistening pearl: Just go."
Pamela R.

———————

When it comes to healthy eating and negative thoughts, you have to be strong for yourself. There may be times when you give in to the cravings, but this should not be all the time. You have to be able to tell yourself, "I am not going to eat [fries] today. I can wait to eat this for my free meal." Another way to get through the negative thought of eating unhealthy food is to always bring your own food not matter where you go.

If you are going to take this journey seriously, there are going to be days where you aren't going to be able to go out to eat with your co-workers, or you may not be able to eat the pie your mother bought. If they pressure you, you can always tell them, "Maybe next time." Don't feel bad about not eating off your plan. Sometimes someone will say, "You've been doing good for a long time, you should reward yourself." This will put negative thoughts in your mind and if you give into them, you will feel guilty later about eating unhealthy food.

Here are some things to remember when it comes to negative thinking:

1. Replace negative thinking with positive thinking.
2. The more you say something, the more you will believe it and then you will do it. If you are always saying, "I can't eat well," you will begin to believe it, then you will stop eating healthfully or not try. But if you say, "I can eat healthy food," and you say it all the time, you will begin to believe it and do it.
3. Remove negative people from your life. You have enough stress with trying to change your own negative thoughts, without other people being negative around you. You need people around you who will encourage you to continue with your journey.
4. Find a support group. There are a lot of great groups out there, with people in it to motivate you and to encourage you to keep going. There are groups on Meetup, Facebook and on many other social networking websites.
5. Remember: For every negative thought, there is a positive one, so don't minimize the positive.
6. Don't speak negatively about other people.
7. Don't make stuff up and believe it. Sometimes we will make things up that aren't true about ourselves or our current situation. No matter what happens to you in life, look at the

positive of it, but don't lie to yourself about reality.

8. Learn to love yourself no matter what you look like. You are a work in progress and this is not going to happen overnight. If you love yourself, you will not put yourself down. Would you tell a child they couldn't do something? No, you would encourage them to do the best they could. Why not treat yourself that way?

9. Make sure you get 7-8 hours of sleep. Not getting enough sleep can encourage negativity. You end up "too tired" to work out, but then you find yourself awake in bed for hours. That one hour when you could have worked out, you were sitting on the couch watching TV feeling sorry for yourself.

10. Don't play the victim, or blame someone else for what you know you should have done. This is your healthy lifestyle journey, no one else's. If you allow someone to take you off your journey, it isn't their fault, it is your fault. I like to tell people, "You make your own decisions and you have to live with the consequences of those decisions. Sometimes the consequences are good and sometimes they are bad, but it comes from the choice you made. Don't let others dictate your choices."

""It's not easy being me but I sure like trying" Johnny L. (This means at some point in life you have to recognize that you are a unique individual and embrace what you have. Once you know recognize your flaws and gifts only then can you be that imperfection constantly striving for perfection. Enjoy the journey to that destination you can see clearly but never reach. Because if you do there's not much reason for others to follow you.)

Chapter 4
Community, Social Media & Weight Loss

After considering the way you think about yourself or your journey, you have to also consider how your community (friends, acquaintances, family, coworkers, people in your city, state, country) can and does affect your ability to find success on a healthy lifestyle journey.

What does community mean to you? According to Merriam-Webster.com, a community is, "a unified body of individuals: as

A. the people with common interests living in a particular area; broadly: the area itself
B. an interacting population of various kinds of individuals (as species) in a common location
C. a group of people with a common characteristic or interest living together within a larger society

Community to me means a group of individuals with the same interest and goals. I can go to the community and ask questions, get motivation, encouragement and advice. In the community there are people living the lifestyle I want to live or they are where I want to be.

"Natural diamonds are created under intense pressure & heat- Be willing to experience your trials with Grace, so you too can come out flawless & tougher than ever" Tabatha "Gigi" W.

Think about the communities you are a part of. What do these communities look like? What benefits are you receiving from the communities? Do you need to be a part of a different community? Are these communities helping you to reach your goals or are these communities holding you back?

When it comes to living a healthy lifestyle you want to be a part of a great community of like-minded people. The health and fitness communities I am a part of I am happy to be a member of (I discuss the communities I am a part of later in this chapter). The communities I am a part of are very supportive, give great free advice and also encourage everyone to keep going. I can post a question to the group and I know at least one person will reply. To give you an example of one of the benefit of being a part of a great community, someone posted the following in one of the fitness and health communities I am a member of. The person posted a picture of her stomach and wanted to know how to get rid of it. This person works out daily, doesn't eat beef and takes in minimum carbs. This person wanted to know what else to do. There were 80 responses to this post. All of the posts were great posts. A lot of great advice and where to start. There was advice from seeing a doctor to doing a cleanse. You may think, there was so many choices how do you make the best choice? Personally, I would start with visiting the doctor because there may be an underlying issue. But the benefit of being in a great community is that you get great advice and you can ask more questions or pick and choose which advice to take.

———◆———

"No matter what you're going through in life, you will always have time to give your body some attention"
Kenroy G.

———◆———

This community has individuals that are personal trainers, beginners, fitness gurus, body builders and those that have reached their goals or are maintaining where they are. What better community to be in. One that's well rounded and that will make you feel welcomed. When you are a part of a community you should never feel out of place.

As modern people, one of the greatest communities we have now is online. Whatever community you decide to be a part of, make sure the community is benefiting you. I believe the more you can contribute to the community the more successful you can be on this healthy lifestyle journey. Before we get into the details of eating plans and exercise in the next chapters (we will get there!), I would like to discuss online community, or social media.

———◆———

"No one can do you better than you do" Mishynn S.

———◆———

In the personal journey stories chapter, I am sure you may have noticed that many people began online. In the next section I want to go over the benefits and rules of joining an online community to give your healthy lifestyle journey support and contacts.

Social Media: Online Diet Tool

Everyone has his or her opinions about social media—some people love it and others detest it—but there are a number of great reasons to use social media, including your health. Joining a social media site, group, or app is a great opportunity to for you to get free advice, workouts, support, motivation and meal ideas that will help you on your journey.

There are a number of social media websites you can join to help you on your weight loss journey. The following are ones I personally recommend:

- Fitocracy – Free/Paid (https://www.fitocracy.com/)
- Facebook – Free (http://facebook.com/)
- Pintrest – Free (https://www.pinterest.com/)
- Dietbet – Paid (http://www.dietbetter.com/)
- Extra Pounds – Free (http://www.extrapounds.com/)
- Daily Mile – Free (http://www.dailymile.com/)
- Twitter – Free (https://twitter.com/)
- Traineo – Free (http://traineo.com/)
- Map My Fitness – Free (http://www.mapmyfitness.com/)
- MyMuscle – Free (https://www.mymuscle.com/)
- Konkura – Free (http://www.konkura.com/)

To learn more about each of these social media websites please visit them at the website listed.

"The pavement glistens when you believe."
Pamela R.

How Can Social Media Help Me?

There are different kinds of social media, which can help you in several different ways on your journey to a healthy lifestyle.

Some groups are a great way to get the support you need—you will have access to people that are starting out like you, or have been where you are now. But even those far ahead of you may be looking for support, and you can help them as well with your feedback. As some of you may know from experience, sometimes those around us—family, co-workers, children, friends—are not very supportive, or as supportive as we would like, of our journey. Joining a group of like-minded people, with similar goals and experiences, can provide the extra support and motivation needed, even when those closest to us may not be able, or willing, to supply it.

"Progressive change needs no apology
or applause, just ACTION." Mishynn S.

One thing you should always be able to get is FREE advice. Whether you are just starting out, or have been working out for a while, you should feel comfortable asking questions concerning workouts and healthy eating. If somebody criticizes you, you should report that person to the administrator of the group. If the administrator doesn't handle the situation, you might want to leave the group. But there are many to join, and one will be right for you and your needs.

Social media can also help you to keep your journey going, when you run into boredom, or a plateau, especially in your exercise routine. Specific groups that focus on running, weight lifting, Zumba or other dance classes, yoga, overall fitness, vegan, vegetarian, low-carb, or other aspects of fitness or healthy eating, can be useful for you to investigate new exercises or eating plans to incorporate into your journey. If you want a routine to begin with, or to spice up your current one, you can see what people in these groups may have posted about their workouts or you can ask a question to the group as to what workouts members do for different body parts. Then you can pick and choose when people respond.

"The Results Will Show Up When You Show Up!"
CHarris ~ CHEKnows Wellness,
Fitness & Lifestyle Expert

Netiquette?

There is such a thing as proper manners, even online. Below are some guidelines to follow when using social media:

- Once you join a website or group, or if you follow someone, NEVER post negative comments. You may see progress pictures of people whom you may or may not think look fit, or who do not look how you would like to look. Remember, they have put a lot of work in to get to where they are. Respect their effort. Even the type of "maybe if you did this, you would have better this" comment is negative, even if it feels like you're being helpful. Unless you're their hired trainer, or they ask for advice, don't post any critical comments.
- Post supportively. Give what you would like to receive in return—positive feedback.
- Be an active member. This means posting about what you're doing, how you're feeling, progress, set-backs, etc. Post about

your exercise activity for the day, not for the entire week, once a week.

- That said, don't be an OVER-active member. Don't drown everybody else with posts ten times a day. Definitely don't link your fitness tracker (Nike+, Fitbit, etc.) to your social media websites. Everything you will do will overrun your newsfeed, and maybe annoy the people whose support you need. Instead of posting your stats on Twitter or Facebook, just post them on the tracker's online website.

- Don't "stalk" members. This should be obvious, but it means, do not send members repeated messages if they go unanswered, or if you can tell the person would rather not continue the conversation; do not comment on a person's postings if they ask you to stop; or any other unwanted behavior toward another member.

- Don't set yourself up to get stalked. Don't list your address or the exact location where you are working out unless you know the individual members of a group can be trusted not to show up unexpectedly.

- Don't post uncomplimentary pictures of yourself, or ones you're not comfortable sharing. Just because you're a respectful member of social media (or you should be!) doesn't mean that everyone is. Don't set yourself up to get mean comments, or to worry about what others will say. Make this about learning to focus on what is improving at the moment and capture that.

- Watch your language. Some websites or groups do not want their members to use inappropriate language (i.e. cursing).

- Read the website or group rules. This will let you know what the owner or administrator expects from the members.

- Use correct spelling. What you say is saved forever.

- Everything you post should be about health, wellness or

fitness. Don't muddle the message with posts related to outside topics like politics, religion, member personal attacks, or the like.

- If there are posts you consider offensive, contact the owner or administrator or the website or group. Let the person know your concerns instead of posting negative comments.
- Remove yourself from a website or group if you don't find it is helpful.

"Put your blinders on and run your race"
Tabatha "Gigi" W.

Support Groups

Online support groups are great for helping you stay focused, committed and consistent on your healthy lifestyle journey. When looking for a support group, do your homework. Ask people you know, research groups in your area and related to your interests, and look up groups online and that are associated with gyms, centers, schools, even workplaces. The more you know about a group's goals and what they can offer you, the more successful you will be.

I am going to discuss four support groups where I am an acting member, as I believe this will show how I personally benefit from my membership in them, and of course, how you could benefit from them, or a group similar to them. All of these can be found online, and/or its group Facebook page. And of course, there are many, many more out there for you to find if these are not your "cup of tea." (Or Gatorade, or unsweetened iced tea, or black coffee, or any other healthy drink you may prefer.)

---

*"Sometimes falling flat on your face is exactly where you'll
find the perspective you need to take you further than ever."*
Mishynn S.

Leading by Example

On March 3, 2014, I started Leading by Example, a health and
fitness support group on Facebook. Group members post recipes,
motivational words of encouragement, workouts and healthy eating
tips. This is an open group on Facebook; anyone can join. When
anyone in the group posts a question, I, or others in the group, are
happy to give answers. Being a part of Leading by Example means
that you are never alone, wherever you are in your healthy lifestyle
journey, and that you will have access to resources for health and
wellness information. This group is focused around the fact that our
health and wellness isn't just about our physical weight loss journey,
but also about our emotional and spiritual journeys as well.

This group is filled with people from all over the world. There are
people from the US but also from Germany, Norway and Mexico.
Not only are people from around the world in this group put the
ages range from teens and up. The members of the group are very
friendly and some of them like to joke around but it is a lot of fun.
This is a group you can come to, to get a wealth of information and
the support you need on your journey.

"The pavement is my canvas to create upon." Pamela R.

On the group page you can also find workouts that will take 20-30 minutes of your time. These workouts range from 30 day challenges and workouts others in the group are doing. I also post my personal workouts, both in the gym, outside and at home along with the meals I eat on a daily basis.

I am open about my journey in the group. Just like anyone else, I have good days and bad days when it comes to eating and working out. I am also not as successful as I would like to be when it comes to eating healthy. There are days where I just give into the cravings that I am having. I post when I am having a bad day to remind people that this is a healthy lifestyle journey, and on this journey you are going to have ups and downs, not matter who you are. For example, I was eating health all day long, when I got home I had a craving for something sweet. I tried to fight it but I lost and ate some candy. Sometimes this happens. I didn't beat myself up about it, I fixed a big bowl of salad with chicken breast and ate it for dinner.

The biggest thing I share with the group is that when you fall down, you need to get back up. Our lives are one big journey. When we hit a bumpy road or when things get tough in life, we don't give up. We find a way to get back on track. This is the same attitude you have to have about your healthy lifestyle journey, and a group like Leading by Example can be one of the tools you use to motivate yourself to drink more water, eat more vegetables, exercise more, to eat healthy again after a night of pizza and beer, or whatever your goals are.

"There is no way to fitness, fitness is the way."
Malgorzata Ch.

If you are interested in joining the Leading by Example Facebook group page, search for Leading By Example (open group) or by typing in https://www.facebook.com/groups/leadingbyexample/ in your web browser.

I also have a great website you can go to for motivation, recipes and workouts. I write a new blog post 2-3 days a week to keep you motivated and encouraged. On the website you will also find a services area. In this area, you will find a list of personal trainers to help you on your healthy lifestyle journey. You can also sign up for workshops, seminars and webinars I will be conducting. To visit my website, go http://www.leadingbyexample.us.

Tiffany Rothe Workouts

Tiffany Rothe has two Facebook pages you can join for support, Tiffany Rothe Workouts (free) and Tiffany Rothe FitClub (paid).

Tiffany Rothe Workouts is a place for fitness inspiration, information and motivation. Her workout routines to help you get Fit, Fierce and Fabulous forever. The goal of her free Facebook page is to help you live the life of your dreams. Working out is the key to unlock the door of your life potential. We are your "go to" directory to help you look better, feel better, eat better, be better.

The Tiffany Rothe FitClub Facebook page is a private group. If you decide to purchase a membership to the Tiffany Rothe FitClub (TRFC), Tiffany will add you to the group page. This page is a place for fitness inspiration, information and motivation. She also supplies free workout routines and 30 day challenges to help you get fit and healthy. Her workouts are a way of life. Her goal is to help you live the life of your dreams. This group is your "go to" directory to help you look, feel, eat and be better.

———— ◈ ————

*"Three pearls to rely upon: Clean food,
clean water and clean health." Pamela R.*

———— ◈ ————

Tiffany answers questions and also gives you suggestions on what you should eat. She, as well as the other members of the group page, will encourage and support you. One day I posted that I did not eat according to the meal plan. I was just being honest about the day I was having. The members of the group came to my rescue. What did they do? They posted encouraging words like, "It's okay, just get back up and get back on track." "You are doing great." I don't know about any of you reading this, but this is the kind of encouragement I need if I get off track. People who are there to lift me up and to help me get back on track.

When you join the Tiffany Rothe FitClub, Tiffany provides each member with a workout schedule and a proven meal plan. Her workouts are made to do anywhere and on your own schedule. Tiffany's effective techniques reduce fat and create toned muscles. You will not count calories or weigh your food as a part of this program, but you will see a noticeable difference in your mid-section after one week. She supplies you with new workouts every week that will keep your body challenged, and with daily inspiration and motivation that will keep your mind engaged.

One of the best things about Tiffany Rothe FitClub, besides the workout and eating plan, is the great support you receive. Everyone goes through the same process when they start no matter how much they weigh, and we all meet the same roadblocks. If you miss a workout, eat fried chicken (when you haven't planned it into your meal schedule), gain 1-2 pounds, or just feel frustrated that you didn't eat according to plan, you can post all this to the group and you will not be judged, but instead find encouragement and motivation to get back on track.

———◦———

"Through all the obstacles, you can do it!!
Just believe in yourself and keep going." Merna B.

———◦———

No matter what is going on in your life, when you post to the group someone will respond with positive words to keep you going. I like to tell everyone who joins, "If you work for the plan, it will work for you."

On Tiffany Rothe FitClub website, Tiffany supplies you with a free workout schedule. You don't have to join the Tiffany Rothe FitClub to receive the free workout. Once on the Tiffany Rothe FitClub home page, click FREE WORKOUT SCHEDULE.

To join Tiffany Rothe workouts – Get In Shape with Online Fitness on Facebook, search for the group name on Facebook or go to https://www.facebook.com/TiffanyRotheWorkouts

To join the Tiffany Rothe FitClub, go to https://www.TRFC.club/.

———◦———

"To be successful, one first must be willing to not just try,
but willing to fail- most success stories began as failed
attempts" Tabatha "Gigi" W.

———◦———

African Americans Over 40, Fit & Fine Group

This group isn't just for African Americans but has welcomed many other nationalities and races to join. This name comes from the creation of the group to promote awareness of health issues that plague the African American community over the age of 40 and to promote helpful information. The founder of this group chose the name "African Americans Over 40 Fit & Fine" because African Americans have the highest rate of obesity, high blood pressure, and diabetes.

This group does not tolerate members who ridicule, belittle or make condescending remarks about other members, or those who use profanity to get their points across. As well, members who "stalk" other members, who post inappropriate comments (including pictures) will be removed from the group. This group is an excellent source of knowledge for living a healthy lifestyle—members range from beginners, trainers, those who compete in fitness competitions, and those who are just living a healthy lifestyle.

"Too many people fall short because their ego is too proud to reach." Mishynn S.

This is a secret group, so the only way you can join is if an existing member adds you. If you are serious about living a healthy lifestyle and want to join this group, contact me on Facebook. I will add you, but your membership will have to be approved by the administrator of the group to become official.

As a member of this group you will get tips both from qualified personal trainers and from regular people who have been on this journey for a while. If you are vegan or vegetarian you will also fit into this group. You will see meals posted by vegans, vegetarians and meat eaters, but every meal posted is healthy and "clean."

If you are concerned about health and fitness for yourself and anyone of any ethnic background that you love, encourage them to join the group with you. Once in the group, you can share your healthy meal plans, workout routines and overall healthy lifestyle so they may be a benefit to others as they were a benefit to you.

"Turn back on your negative thoughts, fears, worries and doubts, and just walk away with your head up and heart full of faith and hope for the best." Malgorzata Ch.

Chapter 5

Understanding What You Should Be and Should Not Be Eating, When, and Why

O k, so you have your mind right, you've looked for a community to help you along, and you're ready to start planning your eating and exercise plans. Let's begin with the basics of eating well. This will be the next most important habit for you in your healthy lifestyle journey, after mind and community.

Before you begin

Before you change your diet, please consult with your doctor. You may need to be on a special diet due to your current health status. If this is the case, please follow the plan your doctor gives you and as your health improves, begin to incorporate the information I provide in this chapter.

———◈———

"It should be considered clean eating if it can fished from the sea, plucked from the ground, has wings to fly or walks on all fours, if not, it should be considered less frequently" Tabatha "Gigi" W.

———◈———

What is Clean Eating?

You may or may not have heard the term "clean eating." Clean eating has been around for years. As society becomes more health-conscious, the more people have started to hear these words. What exactly is "clean eating"? According to Clean Eating Magazine (Team, n.d.), "The soul of clean eating is consuming food in its most natural state, or as close to it as possible. It is not a diet; it's a life-style approach to food and its preparation, leading to an improved life – one meal at a time." When eating "clean" you don't want to eat processed foods, refined sugars, fried foods, soda (or pop, depending on where you are from, this includes diet), and canned foods. Limit the amount of white and wheat products like flour, bread and pasta. I will talk about why you should limit the amount of wheat products later. Now you may be asking, "Well what can I eat?"

When it comes to eating "clean" foods, you want to eat fresh fruits, vegetables (not canned), organic lean meats, healthy fats like avocado and nuts, and foods that are in season. You should drink herbal tea and lots of water. Shop at farmer's markets when possible, and get the entire family involved in eating well. To avoid eating unhealthy food, buy a cooler and pack it with "clean" foods. When you take your cooler with you, this will help you to avoid stopping at fast food restaurants when you are hungry. When you get hungry and you are out by yourself or with you family, you can now open your cooler and eat what you have packed.

"You are the first person to talk to every morning and the last person you talk to every night. And in those soft, quiet moments in your head, you can either lift yourself up or tear yourself down so be mindful of your self-talk." See Jane Sweat

---

What are Carbohydrates (Carbs)?

First, it is okay for you to eat carbs. One of the most important functions that carbs play is to serve as the main energy source or fuel for your body. There are three categories: simple starchy, complex starchy and complex fibrous carbs. You do want to limit the amount of simple carbs you eat, but not all simple carbs are bad for you.

Many natural simple carbs are healthy. These include milk, fruits and some vegetables. These are healthy simple carbs because they are rich in vitamins, minerals and fiber. The bad simple carbs include desserts, candy, soda and sugary cereals. Make sure you limit these.

Complex starchy carbs are found in fruits, vegetables, whole grains, nuts, beans and legumes. Some examples of complex carbs are oatmeal, potatoes, yams, sweet potato, brown rice, whole wheat pasta, whole wheat/multi grain bread, whole grain cereals, whole barley, buckwheat, rye, millet, whole grains, black eyed peas, lentils, chick peas, sweet corn (buy NON GMO) and whole wheat flour.

Complex fibrous carbs include asparagus, eggplant, bamboo shoots, green beans, broccoli, Brussels sprouts, cabbage, carrots, cauliflower, celery cucumber, lettuce, mushrooms, okra, red and green peppers, spinach and zucchini, among others.

Here are some quick facts to keep in mind when it comes to carbs: Brown or green is good for you to eat (whole wheat bread, sweet potatoes, brown rice) and white is bad for you to eat (white bread, white pasta, white potatoes, white rice). Cauliflower is the exception to the rule when it comes to white, as a fibrous vegetable. We will talk later about the timing of eating carbs, but for now let's look at a list of carbs you should eat.

———◦◉◦———

"You are worth the hard work and commitment" John W.

———◦◉◦———

Fruits, Vegetables and Herbs

Below is a list of fruits, vegetables, herbs and other items you can eat. There are many more fruits and vegetables than listed, but this will get you started.

Did you know there are fruit combinations you shouldn't eat together? Sub-acid fruit (apples, pears, peaches, apricot, berries, cherries, grapes, mango, plum) should be eaten with acid fruit (Lime, strawberry, tomato, kiwi, lemons, grapefruit, pineapple, pomegranate). Sub-acid fruit can and should be eaten with sweet fruit (bananas, dates, dried fruits, grapes, papaya, persimmon). But acid fruit doesn't digest well with sweet fruit, so don't mix, for example, bananas and strawberries. Melons digest quickly and should not be mixed with any other fruit.

———◦◉◦———

"YOU Be The Change"!!! Casaline W.

———◦◉◦———

Almonds

Apples

Apricots

Artichoke

Asparagus

Avocado

Balsamic Vinegar

Banana

Basil

Beets

Bell peppers

Blackberries

Blueberries

Boneless/skinless chicken breast

Broccoli

Brown rice

Brown sugar

Brussels sprouts

Canned tuna (in water)

Carrots

Cashews

Cauliflower

Chia seeds

Chili powder

Chive

Cinnamon

Coconut Oil

Coffee (no cream/sugar)

Cucumber

Curry powder

Dark chocolate

Eggs

Fish Oil

Flaxseed/flaxseed oil

Garlic

Ginger

Grapefruit

Green beans

Green tea bags

Hazelnuts

Honey

Jicama

Kale

Leafy greens like arugula

Lean ground turkey

Lemon

Lemons (for water & fish)

Lentils

Lime

Mackerel

Mango

Melons (any kind)

Mrs. Dash seasoning

Multi-vitamins

Mustard

Natural peanut butter or almond butter (ingredient should read only peanuts or almonds, there should be oil on top, low/no sodium).

Oats

Old-fashioned oatmeal (Gluten-free options available)

Olive oil

Onions, leeks, shallots
Oranges
Pam non-stick cooking spray
Pears
Pecans
Pistachio
Plain nonfat Greek yogurt
Pomegranates
Quinoa (Gluten-free options available)
Raspberries
Rosemary
Salmon
Salsa
Spinach
Squash
Stevia
Strawberries
Sweet potatoes
Tangerines
Tilapia
Tofu (Vegan friendly)
Tomatoes
Turmeric
Unsweetened almond milk
Unsweetened baking cocoa
Unsweetened coconut milk
Walnuts
Water
White button mushrooms
Whole wheat bread (Gluten-free options available, I personally use Ezekiel bread)
Wild Salmon
Yam
Zucchini

When Should You Eat Carbs?

There are specific times for eating simple, complex and fibrous carbs. Just as a reminder, carbs help to fuel your muscle tissue growth and recovery, boost your energy, and satisfy hunger and cravings. However, eating carbs at the wrong time encourages your body to store fat, which nobody wants. When are the wrong times, and when are the right times?

Simple carbs such as sugar, honey, and molasses should be eaten before a workout to help supply you with energy and also after your workouts to restock muscle glycogen. If you are eating these carbs at any other time during the day, they promote body-fat storage by increasing insulin release. You want to eat about 25 grams of simple carbs before and/or after an intense workout. Avoid them at any other time during the day.

———◦◉◦———

"Your mind can be your biggest fan or your loudest heckler, keep it in check!" Mishynn S.

———◦◉◦———

Complex carbs such as yams, oatmeal, buckwheat pancakes and brown rice provide your body with slow burning energy without spiking your insulin. Do not eat these carbs around the time of your workout because they provide less immediate energy and slow the absorption of protein into your body. Eat them early in the day. You want to limit or abstain from them in the evenings, when you are less active, because they are more likely to be moved into fat storage rather than burned as energy for your daily movements.

Fibrous carbs such as vegetables, fruits, beans and lentils are high in fiber and have less impact on insulin release. They support gut health and deliver crucial nutrients. Again, you don't want to eat them 1 hour before or 30 minutes after your workout because they slow the absorption of protein into the body. You want to eat several servings a day with an emphasis on vegetables over other carbs later in the day to reduce insulin impact.

Clean Eating Grocery List

Now that we've discussed carbs, it's time to move on to all the rest of the food you need to eat. One of the keys to successful healthy living is knowing what to buy from the grocery store. There are a number of different lists on the Internet, but here is a solid healthy grocery list. I have added this grocery list to the appendix in case you would like to tear it out and take it with you to the store. Happy shopping.

"Learn and grow all you can; Serve and befriend all you can; Enrich and inspire all you can." Eman A.

Fruit	Grains/Beans
Any fruit in season	Black beans (not canned)
Apples	Black bean spaghetti
Avocado	Brown rice
Banana	Brown rice spaghetti
Blackberries	Buckwheat
Blueberries	Cannelini beans (not canned)
Cherries	Chickpeas
Grapefruit	Garbanzo beans
Grapes	Kidney beans
Kiwi	Lentils
Lemons	Lima beans (not canned)
Limes	Millet
Mango	Navy beans (not canned)
Nectarines	Steel-cut oats
Papaya	Peas
Peach	Pinto beans (not canned)
Pears	Quinoa
Pineapple	Tahini
Plums	Tempeh
Pomegranates	
Raspberries	**Sweeteners**
Strawberries	Blackstrap molasses
Watermelon	Local raw honey

Pure maple syrup
Raw dark agave nectar

Meat/Poultry
Albacore tuna (in water)
Beef, grass fed
Bison
Chicken breast
Cod
Eggs
Halibut
Lean ground turkey
Lean ground chicken
Nitrate free bacon (watch the
sodium content)
Salmon, Alaskan
Sardines

Nuts/Seeds
Almonds
Cashews
Chia seeds
Flaxseed
Natural almond butter
Natural peanut butter
Pine nuts
Sunflower seeds
Pecans (raw, no salt)
Pistachios (raw, no salt)
Pumpkin seeds (raw, no salt)
Sesame seeds (raw, no salt)
Sunflower seeds (raw, no salt)

Walnuts (raw, no salt)

Condiments/Oils
Apple cider vinegar
Black pepper
Coconut oil
Extra virgin olive oil
Flaxseed oil
Sesame oil

Liquids
Fruit infused water
Green tea
Herbal tea
Unsweetened coconut milk
Unsweetened almond milk
Water

Herbs - Fresh
Any herbs and spices (not table
salt)
Basil
Cayenne/Chili pepper
Cilantro/parsley
Cinnamon
Cumin
Dill
Ginger
Mint
Mustard seeds
Oregano

Pink Himalayan salt
Red pepper flakes
Rosemary
Thyme
Turmeric

Vegetables
Any vegetable in season
Alfalfa sprouts
Asparagus
Beets

Bok Choy
Broccoli
Brussels sprouts
Cabbage
Carrots
Collard greens
Green beans
Kale
Spinach
Zucchini

Ten Benefits of Drinking Lemon Water

First, use purified water, lukewarm but not scalding hot. Avoid ice-cold water, as that can be difficult for the body to process. It also takes more energy to process ice cold water than the warm. Always use fresh lemons and organic, if possible, never bottled lemon juice.

1. **Aids Digestion.** Lemon juice flushes out unwanted materials and toxins from the body. It encourages the liver to produce bile, an acid required for digestion. Lemons are high in minerals and vitamins and help to loosen toxins in the digestive tract. The digestive qualities of lemon juice help to relieve some symptoms of indigestion, such as heartburn, belching and bloating. The American Cancer Society actually recommends offering warm lemon water to cancer sufferers to help stimulate bowel movements.

2. **Cleanses Your System / is a Diuretic.** Lemon juice helps flush out unwanted materials in part because lemons increase the rate of urination. So toxins are released at a faster rate,

which helps keep the urinary tract healthy.

3. **Boosts Your Immune System.** Lemons are high in vitamin C, which is great for fighting colds. They're also high in potassium, which stimulates brain and nerve function. Potassium also helps control blood pressure. Ascorbic acid (vitamin C) in lemons demonstrates anti-inflammatory effects, and is used as complementary support for asthma and other respiratory symptoms. Plus, it enhances iron absorption in the body.

4. **Balances pH Levels.** Lemons are one of the most alkalizing foods for the body. Sure, they are acidic on their own, but inside our bodies they become alkaline. Disease states only occur when the body pH is acidic. Drinking lemon water regularly can help to remove overall acidity in the body, including uric acid in the joints, which is one of the primary causes of pain and inflammation.

5. **Clears Skin.** The vitamin C component plus other antioxidants helps to decrease wrinkles and blemishes while combatting free radical damage. Vitamin C is vital for healthy glowing skin, while its alkaline nature kills some types of bacteria known to cause acne. It can actually be applied directly to scars or age spots to help reduce their appearance. Since lemon water purges toxins from your blood, the vitamin C contained in the lemon would also be helping to keep your skin clear of blemishes from the inside out.

6. **Energizes You and Enhances Your Mood.** The energy a human receives from food comes not only from the atoms and molecules in your food. The scent of lemon also has mood enhancing and energizing properties. The smell of lemon juice can brighten your mood and help clear your mind. The scent of lemon may also help reduce anxiety and depression.

7. **Promotes Healing.** Ascorbic acid (vitamin C), found in abundance in lemons, promotes wound healing, and is an essential nutrient in the maintenance of healthy bones, connective tissue, and cartilage.

8. **Freshens Breath.** Besides fresher breath, lemons have been known to help relieve tooth pain and gingivitis. Be aware that citric acid can erode tooth enamel, so you should be mindful of this. Do not brush your teeth just after drinking your lemon water. It is best to brush your teeth first, then drink your lemon water, or wait a significant amount of time after drinking to brush your teeth. You can also rinse your mouth with purified water after you finish your lemon water.

9. **Hydrates Your Lymph System.** Warm water and lemon juice supports the immune system by hydrating and replacing fluids lost by your body.

10. **Aids in Weight Loss.** Lemons are high in pectin fiber, which helps fight hunger cravings. Studies have shown people who maintain a more alkaline diet do in fact lose weight faster.

———————

"A meal plan and fitness program are tools, just like a hammer or screwdriver. Unless we pick them up and use them, they're useless. Pick them up!" Jacqueline M.

———————

Beyond the Basics: Cleanses, Additives, GMO's, and Organic

What is a Detox/Body Cleanse?

Detox and cleanse programs focus on the removal of pollutants and toxins (toxins are anything that can potentially harm body tissue) inhaled from the air or absorbed via food or drink. They help with washing out pesticides and chemicals which the body is not naturally equipped to deal with—at the least, they give the body and its organs a break from constantly washing out the junk that the body accumulates. One of the most important functions of a detox or cleanse is to give the body's immune system a break. Our immune systems works overtime whenever we ingest foods that contain or carry harmful chemicals, pesticides, and toxins. Cleanses also impart essential nutrients to the body without chemical additives, large quantities of sugar or sodium, or preservatives. A cleanse can result in increased energy, overall better physical feeling, greater mental clarity, relief of chronic fatigue and/or food intolerances, weight loss and even relief from chronic ill health.

---

*"All of the power you need for living
is stored inside of you." Dr. Verletta S.*

Once a month I do the Mother Nature Cleanse. This cleanse was created by my mentor, Tiffany Rothe. Before beginning a detox or cleanse, make sure you ask the following questions:

1. How does the cleanse work?
2. How will the cleanse effect my body?
3. What is involved in the program?

There are a number of cleanses on the market. Below is a list of some of the different types of detoxes:

- **Chemical:** The body is triggered into cleansing often using herbs or enhanced supplements.
- **Mechanical:** The body is given the opportunity to clean itself, often using fasting and food-based supplements.
- **Colon Cleanse:** Cleans waste from the colon, which may or may not include supplemental products, diet changes, colon irrigation equipment (enema bag, enema board, professional colonic visits).
- **Detox Diet:** Promotes the process of neutralizing or eliminating toxins from the body, most likely will include supplement products, diet changes, and an increase in water intake
- **Heavy Metals Cleanse:** Will cleanse heavy metals from the body, which may or may not include supplemental products, diet changes, colon irrigation equipment, and an increase in water intake.
- **Fasting Cleanse – Type 1 (Avoiding specific foods only):** Requires abstaining from eating certain foods and supplements may be used to maintain nutrition levels.
- **Fasting Cleanse – Type 2 (Avoiding all solid food):** Requires abstaining from all foods, and supplements and/or the juices of certain fruits and/or vegetables may be used to maintain nutrition levels.
- **Fasting Cleanse – Type 3 (No beverages or food):** Requires abstaining from some or all foods and certain beverages (in some, all but water), and supplements may be used to maintain nutrition levels.
- **Non-Fasting Cleanse:** Requires no abstinence from food or beverage.

Don't just go to the store and pick something up. Before beginning a cleanse or detox, do your research. Read online reviews. Ask people you know what cleanses or detoxes they may have done, and what they liked and did not like about them. As stated earlier, I do the Mother Nature Cleanse for five days. During this cleanse, I am drinking warm lemon water every morning, eating only fresh fruits and vegetables, raw nuts, nothing cooked, olive oil and vinegar for salad dressing. If you would like more about this cleanse, you can join Tiffany Rothe's FitClub at www.TRFC.club.

"Bathe in motivation daily. Otherwise you just might have a funky Day." Sherwood G

Additives

Let me start out by saying, I never paid attention to additives in food until after I decided to live a healthy lifestyle. For the first year of my healthy lifestyle, I didn't know the dangers of some additives. I first started researching the facts about additives one year and two months after my journey started. In this section, I will discuss what I have learned about additives, including which ones you should eat and which ones that you should never eat and why. If you are allergic, or have food intolerances, you should always check food labels.

What are Food Additives?

According to the Merriam-Webster dictionary, an additive is "a substance added to another in relatively small amounts to effect a desired change in properties (food additives)." According to dictionary.com, food additives are "substances added directly to food curing or processing, as for preservation, coloring, or stabilizing. It is also something that becomes part of food or affects it as a result of packing or processing as debris or radiation."

———◆———

"Be free... Free of doubt, free of worry and free to live your happiest life being your best you!!!" Brandi W.

———◆———

Food additives are added to foods to:

- Add nutrients
- To help process/prepare food
- Keep products fresh
- Make food appealing

Additives can be man-made or neutral. All products that contain added nutrients must be labeled. Some natural additives are:

- Herbs/spices
- Vinegar, used for pickling foods
- Salt used as a preservative

Some functions of food additives:

- Emulsifiers can prevent food elements from separating
- Stabilizers can provide an even texture
- Anti-caking agents can keep substances flowing freely
- Helping to supply vitamins or nutrients. Many foods are fortified and enriched to provide vitamins, minerals, and other

nutrients that may be low or to lacking in a typical diet or in foods that wouldn't contain them naturally, i.e. flour, cereal, margarine and milk

- Reducing food spoilage that air, fungi, bacteria, or yeast can cause
- Keeping fresh fruit from turning brown when exposed to air
- Helping to change the acid-base balance to achieve a certain flavor or color
- Helping baked goods to rise
- Improving the appearance of food through a certain color
- Helping to bring out the taste in food

"Being fit is much more than physical; it's a mental, emotional, and financial journey. In order to have a fulfilling life all of those aspects have to be in order."
Stephanie M.

Man-Made Additives

Some man-made additives include:

- Antibiotics given to food-producing animals
- Antioxidants in oily or fatty foods
- Artificial sweeteners
- Benzoic acid in fruit juices
- Lecithin, gelatins, corn starch, waxes, gums and propylene glycol in food stabilizers and emulsifiers
- Dyes and coloring substances
- Monosodium glutamate (MSG)

- Nitrates and nitrites in hot dogs and other meat products like lunch meat
- Sulfites in beer, wine and packaged vegetables

I've included an appendix with a list of additives you should and shouldn't eat. I have also included how additives affect your body.

Reading Food Labels and Ingredients

It is very important to pay attention to food and drink labels. One guideline is that you should not drink or eat foods with ingredients in them that you cannot pronounce. The ingredients list should also contain five or less ingredients. Reading labels doesn't just let you know what you are putting in your body, but also what you are feeding your family. You can also make healthier choices once you learn how to read labels and ingredients on drinks and foods.

How do you read Food Nutrition labels?

Start by looking at the serving size and how many servings are in a package. Then check the total calories per serving. Remember that if you eat more than one serving size, you are taking in more calories and nutrients that are listed on the label.

Here is some information to be aware of:

- The information on labels is based on a 2,000 calories a day. Depending on the amount of calories you are eating, you may need to decrease or increase the amount you are eating or drinking.
- For a 2,000 calorie diet, 40 calories per serving is low, 100 calories per serving is moderate and 400 calories or more per serving is high.
- For a 2,000 calorie diet, the total amount of fat per day should

ideally be around 58-78 grams. This should include less than 16 grams of saturated fat and less than 300 mg cholesterol.

- The recommended amount of trans fat is 20 calories or less, which translates to about 2 grams or less.
- If a food label lists 0g trans fat, but does list partially hydrogenated oil in the ingredients, this means there is less than 0.5 grams of trans fat per serving. However, if you eat more than one serving, you could very quickly reach your daily limit of trans fat.

"Being STRONG is a choice you must make DAILY."
Phillip B. IFBB Pro

If a food claims to be...	It means that one serving of the product contains...
Calorie free	Less than 5 calories
Sugar free	Less than 0.5 grams of sugar
Fat	
Fat free	Less than 0.5 grams of fat
Low fat	3 grams of fat or less
Reduced fat or less fat	At least 25 percent less fat than the regular product
Low in saturated fat	1 gram of saturated fat or less, with not more than 15 percent of the calories coming from saturated fat
Lean	Less than 10 grams of fat, 4.5 grams of saturated fat and 95 milligrams of cholesterol
Extra lean	Less than 5 grams of fat, 2 grams of saturated fat and 95 milligrams of cholesterol

Light (Lite)	At least one-third fewer calories or no more than half the fat of the regular product, or no more than half the sodium of the regular product
Cholesterol	
Cholesterol free	Less than 2 milligrams of cholesterol and 2 grams (or less) of saturated fat
Low cholesterol	20 or fewer milligrams of cholesterol and 2 grams or less of saturated fat
Reduced cholesterol	At least 25 percent less cholesterol than the regular product and 2 grams or less of saturated fat
Sodium	
Sodium free or no sodium	Less than 5 milligrams of sodium and no sodium chloride in ingredients
Very low sodium	35 milligrams or less of sodium
Low sodium	140 milligrams or less of sodium
Reduced or less sodium	At least 25 percent less sodium than the regular product
Fiber	
High fiber	5 grams or more of fiber
Good source of fiber	2.5 to 4.9 grams of fiber

Here is an easier way to remember this information:

- "Free" means a food has the least possible amount of the specified nutrient.
- "Very Low" and "Low" means the food has a little more than foods labeled "Free."
- "Reduced" or "Less" mean the food has 25 percent less of a specific nutrient than the regular version of the food.

―――◉―――

"Believe in yourself and your abilities and strengths that you don't know yet you have! Allow yourself the space & time to see what you are truly made of!" Aretha M.

―――◉―――

Food labels can help you limit the amount of sugar, fat and cholesterol you are eating by making it easier for you to compare one food item with another and choose the one with the lower amounts. You can also use food labels to compare how many vitamins, fiber and protein is in foods or drinks. Remember, the information on the food label is based on one serving size. Make sure you understand how much a serving size is when comparing foods and drinks.

Let's look at an example of how to read the label on a bag of chips:

Serving Size: 1 oz (28g/About 11 chips)	
Serving per bag about 3.5	
Calories 140	70 Calories from fat
	% Daily Value
Total Fat 8g	12%
Saturated Fat 1g	6%
Trans Fat 0g	
Cholesterol 0mg	0%
Sodium 210 mg	9%
Total Carbohydrates 16g	5%
Dietary Fiber 1g	4%
Sugar 0 g	
Protein 2g	

People will usually eat this entire bag. The net weight of this bag of chips is 3 3/8 oz (956 g). If you were to eat the entire bag of chips in one sitting you would have consumed:

Calories 490	240 Calories from fat
Total Fat: 28g	42%
Saturated Fat 3.5g	21%
Trans Fat 0g	
Cholesterol 0mg	0%
Sodium 735 mg	31.5%
Total Carbohydrates 56g	17.5%
Dietary Fiber 3.5g	14%
Sugar 0	
Protein 7g	

Ingredients

Just as it important to read the nutrition labels, it is also important to read the ingredients section of all foods.

―――◦◦◦―――

"Bikini bodies are made in the winter." Michelle A

―――◦◦◦―――

Let's look at the same bag of chips, but this time let's look at the ingredients to determine which additives we should and shouldn't be eating:

Ingredient List

Corn, vegetable oil (sunflower, canola, and/or corn oil), maltodextrin (made from corn), salt, cheddar cheese (milk, cheese, cultures, salt, enzymes), whey, monosodium glutamate, buttermilk, Romano cheese (part-skim cow's milk, cheese cultures, salt, enzymes), whey protein concentrate, onion powder, corn flour, natural and artificial flavors, dextrose, tomato powder, lactose, spices, artificial color (including yellow 6, yellow 5, and red 40). Lactic acid, citric acid, sugar, garlic powder, skim milk, red and green bell pepper powder, disodium inosinate, and disodium guanylate.

Some foods are laced with dozens of ingredients with complicated names. When reading ingredients the important thing to remember is that the ingredients are listed in descending order of predominance. The first or three ingredients are the ones that matter most. Ingredients at the bottom of the list may appear in only very tiny amounts.

"If eating healthy is wrong I aint right at all" Nick M.

What ingredients should you look for?

1. The word "whole" such as "whole grain." This should appear as the first or second ingredient. One way to make sure there are whole grains in foods is by looking at the fiber content. Whole grain foods should deliver at least 3 grams of fiber per serving or more.
2. Hidden sugars such as fructose, sucrose and dextrose. A lot of foods contain a lot of sugar, which adds calories without boosting the nutritional value. Words that end in the words

"ose" are all forms of sugar. Other sugars used are honey and corn sweeteners. Four to five grams of sugar is equal to one teaspoon.

3. Partially hydrogenated oils are the primary source of trans-fat. Trans-fats have been known to be more potentially harmful to arteries than saturated fat. Foods that list "trans-fat free" on their package can contain up to ½ a gram of trans-fat per serving.

4. Artificial sweeteners, such as sucralose, saccharin, aspartame and acesulfame. The Center for Science in Public Interest warns that some artificial sweeteners can be dangerous in large quantities. Diet soda (pop) has artificial sweeteners in it.

5. Sodium nitrite and nitrate: These two ingredients are used as a preservative in meats, and can also cause cancer and interact with medications to damage DNA and increase the risk of cancer.

6. Artificial colorings in food: Artificial coloring adds no nutritional value to food. There is research that believes some colorings may pose health dangers. Artificial colorings are often found in cereals, candies, soda (pop) and snack foods.

7. Monosodium Glutamate (MSG): MSG is added to foods to enhance flavor. Some people have experienced the following: headache, flushing, sweating, fluttering heart beat and shortness of breath.

Let's take a look at the ingredients that millions of infants, children and adults drink. We are going to look at the ingredients in cow's milk.

According to Dr. Edward Group III, the founder of the Global Healing Center, due to the extreme processes that milk goes through and the high amounts of antibiotics, hormones, and genetically-modified substances that cows are continually exposed to, there are real and eminent concerns associated with drinking milk from cows. All cows release toxins through their milk, as milk is a natural exit-portal for substances that the body cannot use.

"I make time for me because I'm worth it." Paulina S.

The following ingredients have been added to cow's milk:

1. Hormones: pituitary, steroid, hypothalamic and thyroid hormones.
2. Gastrointestinal Peptides: Nerve and epidermal growth factors
3. rBGH (Recombinant Bovine Growth Hormone): This genetically engineered hormone is directly linked to breast, colon and prostate cancer. This is injected into cows to increase milk production.
4. Pus: National averages show at least 322 million cell-counts of pus per glass! This is well above the human limit for pus-intake, and has been directly linked to paratuberculosis bacteria, as well as Crohn's disease. The pus comes from infected udders on the cows known as mastitis.
5. Blood cells: The USDA allows up to 1.5 million white blood cells per milliliter of commonly-sold milk.
6. Antibiotics: Cows are often in a state of disease and mistreatment and thus are continually being injected with antibiotic medicines, and rubbed down with chemical-laden ointments to deal with their chronic infections. Regulating committees only test for 4 of the 85 drugs in dairy cows. The

other 81 drugs found in cow's milk are being drunk by you, your family and friends.

What is there to drink besides cow's milk? You can drink or add coconut, hazelnut, goat, rice, hemp or almond milk to your foods.

———

*"It's YOUR health!!...DO your BEST
to BE your BEST!!..." Alex K.*

———

Non GMO Foods

Non GMO is another term you may begin to notice on foods or products. A GMO (genetically modified organism) is a plant or animal created through the gene splicing techniques of biotechnology (also called genetic engineering, or GE). This experimental technology merges DNA from different species, creating unstable combinations of plant, animal, bacterial and viral genes that cannot occur in nature or in traditional crossbreeding. The following are high-risk crops:

- **Alfalfa** (first planting 2011)
- **Canola** (approx. 90% of U.S. crop)
- **Corn** (approx. 88% of U.S. crop in 2011)
- **Cotton** (approx. 90% of U.S. crop in 2011)
- **Papaya** (most of Hawaiian crop; approximately 988 acres)
- **Soy** (approx. 94% of U.S. crop in 2011)
- **Sugar Beets** (approx. 95% of U.S. crop in 2010)
- **Zucchini and Yellow Summer Squash** (approx. 25,000 acres)

Monitored Crops (those for which suspected or known incidents of contamination have occurred, and those crops which have genetically modified relatives in commercial production with which cross-pollination is possible.; The Non-GMO Project test regularly to assess risk, and move to "High-Risk" category for ongoing testing if we see contamination):

- *Beta vulgaris* (e.g., chard, table beets)
- *Brassica napa* (e.g., rutabaga, Siberian kale)
- *Brassica rapa* (e.g., bok choy, mizuna, Chinese cabbage, turnip, rapini, tatsoi)
- *Cucurbita* (acorn squash, delicata squash, patty pan)
- Flax
- Rice
- Wheat

———◎———

*"May the gift of Life Nourish
your soul with vitality." Leonard V.*

———◎———

Common Ingredients Derived from GMO Risk Crops

The following ingredients have been derived from GMO at risk crops. This is why it is important to read label on everything:

Amino Acids, Aspartame, Ascorbic Acid, Sodium Ascorbate, Vitamin C, Citric Acid, Sodium Citrate, Ethanol, Flavorings ("natural" and "artificial"), High-Fructose Corn Syrup, Hydrolyzed Vegetable Protein, Lactic Acid, Maltodextrins, Molasses, Monosodium Glutamate, Sucrose, Textured Vegetable Protein (TVP), Xanthan Gum, Vitamins, Yeast Products

More and more products now have the NON-GMO logo on them to let you as a consumer know the food or product is a NON-GMO product. Look for this logo on foods:

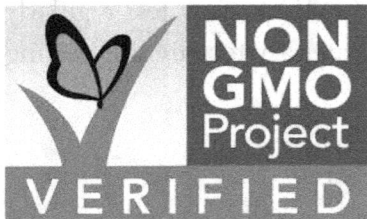

To learn more about NON-GMO foods and products, please visit: http://www.nongmoproject.org/.

Best Way to Avoid GMOs

Both USDA organic certification and the Non-GMO Project seal are great methods for avoiding GMOs. Furthermore, both labels are helping to provide greater transparency for consumers about what's in their food and how it's being produced.

Beyond banning GMOs in fresh and processed organic foods, the USDA organic certification takes a holistic approach to the health of our food system and food producers. Organic products are produced without the use of synthetic chemicals, which are dangerous for farmers, consumers, our land, and our water systems. These extra steps help to promote a sustainable and safe food system.

"Never let your palate control the quality of your life!!!"
Babette D.

The Non-GMO Project's strict set of standards and guidelines, including multi-level testing, ensures that companies and producers are avoiding GMOs in all aspects of production. The Non-GMO Project also provides education to the public about the risks associated with GMOs, the importance of labeling, and tips about how to best avoid them.

Go Organic for Unprocessed Foods

Unfortunately, the Non-GMO Project only verifies meats and processed foods commonly found in the center aisles of the grocery store. Due to the lack of verification for fresh produce, buying certified organic produce is the only way to avoid GMOs in your fresh foods.

Since the US government does not enforce the labeling of GMOs for all food producers, the Non-GMO Project is filling a much-needed void. Choosing any product that has been verified by The Non-GMO Project is a safe bet for avoiding GMOs, and it's the only safeguard against GMOs when not buying organic.

———◉———

"Nutrition is 96% of battle the other 4% is fun Workouts"
John W.

———◉———

Organic Foods

You may also see the following logo on organic foods:

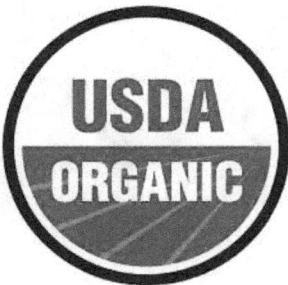

Organic agriculture produces products using methods that preserve the environment and avoid most synthetic materials, such as pesticides and antibiotics. The USDA ORGANIC logo verifies that irradiation, sewage sludge, synthetic fertilizers, prohibited pesticides, and genetically modified organisms were not used in the making of the product. When it comes to livestock, producers met animal health and welfare standards, did not use antibiotics or growth hormones, and used 100% organic feed and provided animals with access to the outdoors. To learn more about organic products, please visit the United States Department of Agriculture websites: http://fnic.nal.usda.gov/food-labeling/organic-foods and http://www.ams.usda.gov/AMSv1.0/NOPOrganicStandards

The Difference Between USDA Organic and Non-GMO Verified Seal

Many consumers are looking for ways to avoid genetically modified organisms (GMOs) in their food. There are currently two food labels that indicate the absence of GMOs for consumers: the USDA Organic label and the Non-GMO Project Verified seal.

As a local supporter of transparency in our food system, I think it's great that consumers are able to make informed decisions about GMOs through both the Non-GMO Project and USDA Organic certification.

What's the difference between these two labels, and what do they mean in terms of GMO avoidance? Here's a general overview of the two labels and their verification processes.

"Success starts with your health because when you're healthy all things are possible" Vincent F.

USDA Certified Organic Seal:

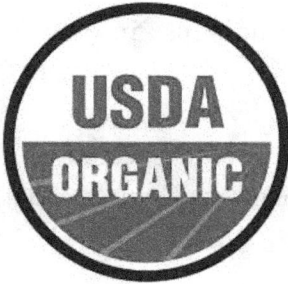

The National Organic Program is regulated by the United States Department of Agriculture (USDA). Their organic certification is a process-based certification that requires farmers and producers to follow approved methods in order to achieve organic certification.

GMOs are prohibited from certified organic products, which means farmers are not allowed to grow produce from GMO seeds, their animals can't eat GMO feed, and organic food producers can't use GMO ingredients.

Certified organic farms and facilities follow a site-specific organic system plan and are inspected annually by third-party organic inspectors to ensure compliance. In order to fulfill the USDA organic regulations, farmers and processors must prove that they aren't using GMOs in any part of their production and are utilizing approved practices to protect their products or crops.

All USDA certified organic produce, grains, meats, and processed foods do not allow the use of GMOs.

"The Journey to good health starts in your mind and is fueled by your hearts desires to be better." Kimberly M.

What does the organic certification mean?

- Processed foods with 95%-100% certified organic ingredients can be certified to use the USDA Organic Seal. The other 5% like salt and water cannot contain GMOs.

- Prohibits use of chemical fertilizers, synthetic substances, irradiation, sewage sludge, or GMOs in organic production.
- Prohibits antibiotic and synthetic hormone use in organic meat and poultry.
- Requires 100% organic feed for organic livestock.
- Verification is maintained through 3rd party inspectors' annual site inspections, organic system plan review, and residue testing.*

*Residue testing is only done when inspectors are concerned that farms or businesses have used prohibited substances or methods. Tests can be random or risk-based, but are not mandatory.

———◦———

"What are you telling your body when you feed it junk? Love yourself enough to fuel your body with nutritious food." Otisa J.

———◦———

The Non-GMO Project's Non-GMO Seal:

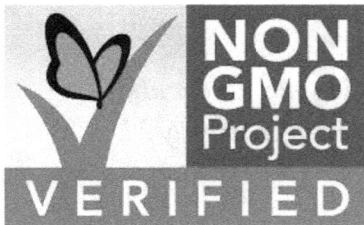

The Non-GMO Project is a non-profit organization that independently offers GMO test verification and labeling for non-GMO products. Their verification is process-based, using traceability, segregation, and testing to ensure compliance with their standards.

Companies looking to receive the Non-GMO Project stamp must follow the project's standards of best practices and have product testing conducted at various stages of production, anywhere from the field to the packaging facility.

Despite their inspection process, the project can't legally claim products to be "GMO free" because the contamination risks to seeds, crops, and ingredients are too high. However, they're the only organization offering independent verification of testing for GMO products in the US and Canada.

———⊙———

"YOU are a rock star! So act like one. Be open to learning and trying new things. When one fitness program or meal plan doesn't interest you find a new one. The goal is to create an enjoyable healthy lifestyle that doesn't feel like a chore. That's what has always worked for me and helps me to maintain results. It starts with having the right mindset. I'm cheering for ya in spirit!" Ebonie A.

———⊙———

What does the Non-GMO Project's Verification Process require?

- Ongoing testing of all at-risk ingredients – any ingredient that is grown commercially in GMO form must be tested prior to use in a verified product.
- An Action Threshold of 0.9%. This is in alignment with laws in the European Union, where any product containing more than 0.9% GMO must be labeled.
- Absence of all GMOs is the target for all Non-GMO Project Standard compliant products. Continuous improvement towards achieving this goal must be part of the Participant's quality management systems.
- After the test, they require rigorous traceability and

segregation practices to be followed in order to ensure ingredient integrity through to the finished product.

- For low-risk ingredients, they conduct a review of ingredient specification sheets to determine absence of GMO risk.
- Verification is maintained through an annual audit, along with onsite inspections for high-risk products.

"We can't CONTINUE to expect CHANGE if we don't continue to TAKE ACTION." Phillip B. IFBB Pro

Key Differences Between the Labels:

Practices	USDA Certified Organic Label	NON-GMO Project Seal
Prohibits use of chemical/synthetic fertilizers and pesticides	X	
Prohibits antibiotic and synthetic hormone use	X	
Regulated by the government (USA)	X	
Mandatory testing for GMOs at multiple levels of production		X
Prohibits GMOs in all aspects of farming and processing	X	X
Trustworthy method to avoid GMOS	X	X

Pesticides on Fruits and Vegetables

According to the Environmental Working Group (EWG), some 65% of thousands of produce samples analyzed by the US

Department of Agriculture test positive for pesticide residues. EWG analyzed pesticide residue testing data from the US Department of Agriculture and Food and Drug Administration to come up with 48 fruits and vegetables with pesticide residue. The list is from worst to best.

1. Apples
2. Strawberries
3. Grapes
4. Celery
5. Peaches
6. Spinach
7. Sweet bell peppers
8. Nectarines – imported
9. Cucumbers
10. Cherry tomatoes
11. Snap peas – imported
12. Potatoes
13. Hot peppers
14. Blueberries – domestic
15. Lettuce
16. Kale/collard greens
17. Plums
18. Cherries
19. Nectarines – domestic
20. Pears
21. Tangerines
22. Carrots
23. Blueberries –imported
24. Green beans
25. Winter squash
26. Summer squash
27. Raspberries
28. Broccoli
29. Snap peas –domestic
30. Green onions
31. Oranges
32. Bananas
33. Tomatoes
34. Watermelon
35. Honeydew melons
36. Mushrooms
37. Sweet potatoes
38. Cauliflower
39. Cantaloupe
40. Grapefruit
41. Eggplant
42. Kiwi
43. Papayas
44. Mangoes
45. Asparagus
46. Onions
47. Sweet peas – frozen
48. Cabbage
49. Pineapples
50. Sweet corn
51. Avocado

The top twelve on the list are known as the "dirty dozen" and the bottom 15 are known as the "clean fifteen." To avoid eating unclean vegetables and fruits, go for the organic version. If you are unable to afford to buy organic vegetables and fruits, make sure you clean them well.

How to Clean Fruits and Vegetables

Smooth-Skinned Produce

Keeping a blend of vinegar and water in a 1 to 3 ratio in a spray bottle makes cleaning smooth-skinned produce easier. Use the spray bottle to mist the fruit or vegetable, thoroughly coating its exterior with the vinegar solution. Allow the produce to rest for 30 seconds before rubbing its surface and rinsing it under cold, running water. This removes all vinegar taste. The FDA recommends cleaning smooth-skinned fruits and vegetables by gently rubbing them with your hands instead of an abrasive scrubber. This prevents you from breaking the skin before the fruit or vegetable is completely clean, which could expose the flesh to contaminants. Tomatoes, apples and grapes are examples of smooth-skinned produce.

"One small step is all that's needed to begin a journey." Chris R.

Rough or Firm-Surfaced Produce

Broccoli, cauliflower, leafy greens, melons, potatoes, berries and other produce without a smooth or soft surface are slightly more difficult to clean. They require a soaking in a 1 to 3 vinegar and water mixture. This ensures the acidic blend kills all bacteria. For heads of cabbage or other greens, you will need to separate the individual leaves for thorough cleaning. This can be a bit impractical at times, but if you use your sink as the container for the water and vinegar mixture, you should have plenty of room. After their soak, scrub the vegetables with a brush and rinse them under running water.

Another way to wash your fruits and vegetables is to fill a large bowl with cold water then add in ¼ cup vinegar and 2 tablespoons salt and swish around with hands. Place the vegetables and fruit in and soak for 30 minutes, soaking will not affect the flavor. Rinse under cold water and dry. The vinegar cleans the fruits and vegetables and the salt will draw out any little bugs and dirt.

You can also do the following to clean your fruits. Fill the sink with water, add 1 cup of vinegar, and stir. Add all fruit, and soak for 10 minutes. The water will be dirty and the fruit will sparkle with no wax or dirty film. This is great for berries also as it will keep them from molding. You can also do this with strawberries, and they will last for weeks.

Washing your fruits and vegetables with vinegar also prevents them from become moldy too quickly. Washing your fruits and vegetables with vinegar doesn't leave them tasting like vinegar! They will now taste like they are supposed to—fresh, clean fruit.

"Being healthy and fit isn't a fad that comes
and goes, it's a lifestyle" Vincent F.

Chapter 6
How to Start Exercising

A nd now that we've discussed mind, community, and eating, let's move on to moving your body.

Before you start any exercise program, please consult with your doctor especially if you haven't exercised in a long time or you have chronic health problems, such as heart disease, diabetes or arthritis, or if you have any other concerns.

Benefits of Exercising

No matter where you start when it comes to exercising, there are great benefits to exercising including weight loss, increased energy and stress relief. It also makes you feel good and look great, it puts you in a good mood and it makes others want to join you, just to name a few.

Exercising can help you from gaining excess weight, to maintain weight loss, or to lose weight. It's simple: When you exercise, you burn calories. The more intense the workout or exercise, the more calories you burn. There are even ways to burn calories if you don't have time to exercise before going to work or after coming home. You can take the stairs, walk around your building, or find a YouTube exercise video to do at your desk.

—◦—

"Comfortable does not equal change." Justina G.

—◦—

Exercise also improves overall health conditions—it helps to lower blood pressure and it also boosts the "good" cholesterol in your body. Exercising can also help to prevent strokes, type II diabetes, depression, certain types of cancers, and arthritis, among others.

I used to play racquet ball with a guy in his twenties like me. He was very muscular, a former college football player, and he would often come to the court for stress release. He would take all his anger and stress out on the ball. If you are in a bad mood or stressed out, getting sweaty in a workout could be a great way for you to feel better. (I have to admit that I did not play with him on the days he was "relieving stress." If you have ever played racquet ball, you know that getting hit with the ball from even a regular swing really hurts. So you could imagine how much pain getting hit with *that* ball would cause!) But please listen to your body. When I am stressed out, I cannot work out. My mind wonders too much and I cannot concentrate on what I am doing. I would rather get my thoughts together, deal with the issue, *then* go to the gym. I don't want to hurt myself thinking about the issue. That would just stress me out further.

—◦—

"Conviction leads to Addiction. #Lifestylechange." Israel M.

—◦—

Physical activity stimulates various brain chemicals that may leave you feeling happier and more relaxed. You may also feel better about your appearance and yourself when you exercise regularly, which can boost your confidence and improve your self-esteem. As I lost weight and began to like what I saw in the mirror, it truly gave me more self-esteem and confidence. I loved the way I looked and how I felt. I didn't walk around cocky, but confident instead. I walked with my head held high and my shoulders back. Let me clear something up before moving on: I have liked the way I look, but not loved it. You should like how you look now; that way, as your body transforms, you will be able to love that transformation.

Exercising on a regular basis can also improve your muscle strength and boost your endurance by delivering oxygen and nutrients to your tissue and helping your cardiovascular system to work more efficiently. Your cardiovascular system consists of your heart and lungs. The stronger your heart and lungs are, the more energy you will have throughout the day.

Most people believe exercise helps you to sleep better, but it can also pep you up. When I exercise in the morning, I can take a shower and go straight to sleep at night, but when I exercise in the evenings, I am unable to sleep through the night. I know other people who have told me that when they exercise, it gives them energy. If you work out a couple of hours before bedtime, when you do go to sleep, exercise can help you to fall asleep faster and go into a deeper sleep. Just make sure you don't exercise too close to bedtime, or you will be up all night like me.

———◦———

"Do not allow others to discourage your ambition and dreams." Dennis R.

———◦———

Whether you exercise with others or by yourself, it can and should be fun. There are so many ways to work exercise into your day, especially if you have children. Just running around chasing them is exercise. When my daughter was younger, I took her to the park and we played and ran all around. I was so tired when I finished playing with her, but it was a great calorie burn.

Did you know that exercise could help you to become more creative? A really good work out can boost creativity for up to two hours after the workout. The next time you need some creativity for a project, take a nice long walk or hike.

Studies show that most people perform better on aerobic tests when they are working out with a partner or in a class. This could be due to the fact we as humans like to compete against others. We don't want someone to outdo us, so we try to keep pace with those around us and tend to push harder than if we had worked out alone. We push each other to walk or run a little further, or to push out a few more reps.

When it comes to exercising and to being successful, do what you love. Try different things. Not everyone likes to lift weights. You may not like lifting weights, but you may like an exercise or fitness class that incorporates weights. Try different fitness classes, running, walking, group exercise, boot camps, dancing, karate, videos, yoga, biking, swimming, etc. to see what you like and start there. The more you like what you are doing, the more successful you will be at doing it.

"Don't be afraid to step out on faith and follow your heart." Cabrini S.

Walking/Running

One of the easiest things you can do is to start walking, and it is free. Some people think that when they start working out, they need to hire a trainer or to go to the gym. But to start out, if you begin walking and make modifications to your diet, the weight will begin to come off.

Walking is a great time to talk to God, reflect on life, enjoy the surroundings, meet new people and have great conversations with friends or family members. You don't have to walk alone, but if you do and you are wearing head phones, please pay attention to your surroundings and walk with one ear covered instead of both to hear what is going on around you.

If you want to walk, but you don't want to walk by yourself, there are walking groups you can join or you can even start your own group. Below are two groups I can suggest if you would like to start walking in a group.

Sisters in Health and Fitness Walking Group

This organization is always looking for people to start a walking group in different cities. If you would like to start a walking group in your city, or if you would like to find out about a walking group in your city, please send Sandi an email at info@sifh-wellness.com or visit her website to learn more about the walking groups. http://sifh-wellness.com/about-sifh/latesthappenings/walking-groups/

"It's All About the JOURNEY" Sandi J

Black Girls Run

Black Girls Run has a number of walk/run groups throughout the United States. Anyone can join this group. There are many ladies of different races participating in the group. If you would like to join one of their groups, please visit their website at www.blackgirlsrun. com or find them on Facebook.

If you become a member of a running group on social media, see if there are people who live in your area or if there is a chapter or the running group in your area. This is a great way to get out and run with other people like yourself. Running groups have people in them that are beginning or those that are running marathons. If you are just starting out, you will fit into the running group.

———————

"Don't look for the journey to be easy. You're going to have to put yourself on the other side of fear to make it happen. You'll make mistakes and even get upset, but just don't QUIT!" Charles M.

———————

Ree & Rhonni's Walking Group

Ree & Rhonni's Walking Group of St. Louis, Missouri was started in June 2014 by Aretha (Ree) McFall & LaRhonda (Rhonni) Larthridge.

The need to start some type of fitness group had been a vision of mine since 2011 but fear kept me from it. I didn't know where to start and I feared that no one would support it!

The goal was to target members in need – men, women and children who were faced with health issues as a result of inactivity and who were also struggling to change their lifestyle. I understood that the struggles can be for a myriad of reasons; their current physical condition may make the prospect of joining a gym very intimidating, economics may be a barrier, they may have little to no wellness knowledge and have no idea where to start, or they may be so unhappy with their physical state that they have simply given up.

In 2014, when I received an invite from a friend on Facebook to become a local walking group leader that would represent a National Chapter called Sisters in Fitness an d Health, I jumped at the opportunity! This is when I realized this was definitely a sign and that I was supposed to be living my dream of impacting the lives of those in my community & making a difference through fitness & health.

"If you want something different, not only do you have to do something different, but you have to change your mind and go in another direction!" Aretha M.

I needed a second lieutenant who would be just as committed as I was and who would back me up and always show up even if I couldn't to support, motivate and encourage the group and I couldn't have chosen a better person that my sister Rhonni! She is physically active, a great motivator and so very creative. She encourages the group to constantly challenge themselves. I LOVE her to the moon and back and so does our group.

We chose a central location, the St. Louis Gateway Arch ground which is a National Monument and a location that would attract many people due to its location and serene environment. We also decided Tuesdays at 6:30 p.m. and Saturday Mornings at 8:00 a.m. would fit most people's schedules.

Our walks are usually no more than an hour, with a minimum

of 3 miles which includes mini hills. However, for those just starting out and that have physical limitations, we have cut off points approximately every ½ mile and there's also a track available for those who don't care to walk the perimeter. Our group is unique because while Rhonni leads the group for those who walk at a faster pace or for those who like a little more challenge and like to run, I bring up the rear to ensure those who need a slower pace or who might struggle make it to the finish line. When we say we leave no one behind, we mean just that. If they have the time, we have the time!

We welcome everyone; women, men and children are encouraged to come regardless of your physical conditioning.

"Don't stagnate Accelerate" Leonard V.

Our Mottos are:

- Take that 1st step, we promise you won't regret it!
- One Step, One Day at a Time towards One Goal!
- We leave no one behind
- We will meet you where you are!

Many of our novice walkers simply cannot believe that we show up for them twice a week every week to encourage them, inspire them and to walk alongside them right through their struggle to the finish line.

If you would like to start your own group, it doesn't require much. Spread the word, get organized — before you know it, you and your group are taking steps together toward better health. Here are some strategies to get started.

How to Create a Walking Group

1. **Create a flier to announce your meeting.** Include time, location and a telephone number if you don't mind taking calls. You might post your flier at these locations:

    *   Mall
    *   Post office
    *   Church, mosque, synagogue or temple
    *   Community center
    *   Workplace
    *   Health club
    *   Senior center

    Besides posting a flier, consider advertising in your local newspaper, workplace classified ads or on a community (example Meet Up) or social networking website site.

    Consider holding the meeting at a public location such as the local library or community center—that way you don't have to worry about inviting strangers into your home.

"Don't think or talk about it. Just put on your shoes and DO it!" Heike F.

---

2. **Get organized at your first meeting.** Warmly greet all potential members of the group and request that everyone wear a name tag. Ask guests to provide their name, address, phone number and e-mail address so that you can contact them about upcoming events. Then get down to business to discuss:

- How often to walk
- The time of day and days of the week to meet
- Most convenient locations to meet
- What route(s) to take
- The distance you plan to cover
- The time you plan to spend per walk
    You may want to get more organized as the momentum of your group builds. Examples include:
- Deciding on a name for your group and designing a team logo
- Developing a newsletter
- Entering charity walking events as a group
- Competing with other walking groups for distance walked or money raised for charity
    Group members may have more ideas, too.

———◆———

"Dreams are concocted by the mind for one's pleasure, but goals are achieved through hard work." Dana G

———◆———

3. **Maintain your group's momentum.** As the group leader, encourage the group to have a motivational meeting at least once a month. Motivational activities may include:

- Inviting a guest speaker to discusses health and fitness
- Sharing stories about how walking affects your physical and mental health
- Welcoming new members
- Celebrating the success of the group
    The best bet is to ask the group what sort of activities

would inspire and motivate them and get them involved in making those activities happen.

4. **Enjoy yourself.** The camaraderie you experience in a walking group can help you stay on track with walking for fitness. And the new friends you make can make it well worth the effort.

Walking/Running Shoes

Once, my sister took my dad to a running store because he said the walking shoes he bought were too small, but his feet couldn't have grown because he has worn the same size for years.

At the store, a salesperson explained to him that when you walk (or run), you need to make sure you buy walking (or running) shoes. When you walk (or run) your feet expand in different ways, and each specific type of shoe is made for your feet to expand in a specific way. He also found out that his feet actually did grow ½ inch. Because of all of the walking he was doing, his arch had started to fall and this was the cause of his foot growing.

Invest in a great pair of gym shoes. Better yet, go to a running store and have them do a gait analysis. A gait analysis is when a clerk at your local running store watches you jog, and suggests a pair of shoes that are more stable, or more neutral, or more cushioned, or a pair that "forces" you to land mid-foot. When you are analyzed statically (standing), dynamically (moving), as well as when running on a treadmill during a gait analysis, it serves to provide a unique, personal movement "map." That "map" reveals the programming of everything happening within your body—from kinesthetic awareness and habit, to individual levels of mobility, stability, flexibility, and functional strength. The analysis of all these different elements taken together is what creates a complete picture of a person's gait. In essence, it is far more than just gait analysis. It is a true "movement" analysis.

―――⟨◉⟩―――

"Don't wish. Work." Paulina S.

―――⟨◉⟩―――

Gait analysis uncovers precisely how your body is moving. Every activity, even standing still, represents a unique movement pattern. That pattern is bred from your habits and lifestyle, as well as your body's mobility, stability, flexibility and strength. Every action you take—running stride, pedal stroke, swim stroke, etc.—represents that unique movement pattern. If your movements include compensations (and they likely do), gait analysis can pinpoint the areas in the body where these losses of efficiency originate.

Some walking/running injuries come from the body compensating; the larger muscles in the body, hamstrings, glutes, quads, etc. become less active and end up contributing less to the body's movement. This leads the smaller or tiny stabilizing muscles to step in, or compensate, and do the work of the larger muscles. These smaller muscles over time sustain a lot of wear and tear, which can cause injuries.

―――⟨◉⟩―――

"Exercise to be functional. Eat to nourish your cells. Drink to stay hydrated. BREATHE DEEPLY the breath of life."
Sherwood G

―――⟨◉⟩―――

Fitness shoes are expensive, but you can ask for last year's model. If they were the top shoes last year, they will still work for you a year later and they may be a lot cheaper.

Walking/running can also affect your ankles, shins, knees and hips. This is another reason to make sure you are wearing a great shoe. You want to buy a new pair every 6 months or 300-400 miles. If you need to, also invest in arch support.

Personal Trainer

When hiring a personal trainer please do your research. Remember: Don't hire the cheapest person you can find, and not every personal trainer is right for you. Below is a list of questions to ask a personal trainer. I have also answered some of these questions for you.

How do you stay in shape? This question allows you to see what exercises and what the person may suggest you do if you are able to do them.

What's your fitness philosophy? Every personal trainer should tell you what he/she believes when it comes to fitness. This question allows you to see the type of goals the personal trainer has for his/her clients. For example, are they training their clients for better health or more confidence? To be in better shape, or to train for competitions?

"Fitness is yours. Own it." Paulina S.

Do you recommend supplements? This is not a question personal trainers should be answering because it is out of their scope of practice unless they are a registered dietitian. Please be careful of taking supplements that just anyone suggests, without first speaking to your doctor and researching the supplements.

Are you CPR and AED certified? AED stands for automated external defibrillator and if you or someone else at the gym has a heart attack, it can save a life. Make sure your personal trainer knows how to use it and is properly trained to respond during potential emergencies.

Are most of your clients long term or short term? If a personal trainer has mostly long-term clients, then you know that he or she is probably good at relationship building and at keeping workouts fresh and challenging over time. On the flip side, if they're all short-term, this might signify that the personal trainer is either brand new to the industry (you should definitely ask about previous training experience) or a fitness facility. At worst, this could signal an underlying training or personality issue.

A lot of personal trainers, train as a part-time job, so if this number is below 10, don't be afraid. Just follow up by asking whether they have a full-time job. If they don't have another job, it is okay for you to ask why they train so infrequently. If they do 30-plus sessions a week, ask them how they keep things fresh and how they avoid burnout.

"Fitness starts in the mind then spreads throughout the body."
Vincent F.

Why are you a personal trainer? Similar to, but different from, question No. 2, this one addresses why the trainer got into the fitness field. If it's to see people transform their bodies, then you know the trainer focuses on the physical. If the trainer says it's to help people transform their lives, then you know they'll probably have your well-being in mind.

How many days per week do I need to work out? This depending on your health and fitness goals. The personal trainer should go over this with you and let you know what will work best for you.

What should I eat before a workout? Ideally, you should have some form of fuel in your system before you work out. The personal trainer can advise you on what you should eat before you work out.

What should I eat after a workout? Eating after a workout is important. You need to replenish your glycogen stores and 'feed' the muscles that you've just trained.

What are the best exercises for getting rid of muffin tops/bat wings/inner thigh bulge? Excess fat on the belly, upper arms and inner thighs doesn't typically occur in isolation. If you've got it there, chances are you've got it everywhere. You can't spot reduce. No exercise will target fat cells in just one part of the body. You need to target them all via exercise and proper nutrition.

And if you really want to see muscle definition once the layer of subcutaneous fat is shed, make sure you're following a strength training program designed for muscular hypertrophy. (Here's where having a personal trainer comes in handy.)

"Go for it and try. If you fail at least you know what not to do the next time." Cabrini S.

Why can't I just do cardio? While cardiovascular training is great for building strong hearts and lungs, it doesn't provide the stimulus your body needs to build bigger, stronger muscles and bones.

How quickly will I see the results of my training? Expect to FEEL the results of your training sooner than you SEE them.

What's the best diet for weight loss? Any meal plan you can stick with for as long as it's going to take. Studies have shown that regardless of the diet followed, adherence is the only thing that predicts success. Beware of any diet that promises rapid weight loss (and expects you to consume fewer than 1,000 calories per day.)

*"Gratitude for your precious body will make
your journey a miracle." Heike F.*

Are you looking for a personal trainer? Here are a few you can contact:

Israel McGhee
Israel McGee
israelmcghee@hotmail.com
919-940-1700
Facebook.com/mcgheeisrael

Kenroy Grant
Personal Trainer
theworldofdo@gmail.com
404-587-0419
Atlanta, Georgia

During my childhood, I was introduced into the world of holistic health and wellness by my mother. This has been a valuable part of my personal health regimen and one I integrate into my clients' fitness plans. I've motivated people for 28 years with the last 15 as a professional trainer. I've trained a full spectrum of professional clients with different fitness goals and challenges, including:

- Obesity
- Sports Injuries
- Executive Level Stress Management/Work-Life Balance
- Pre/Post-Natal Training

- Weight Loss and Weight Management
- Nutritional Counseling and Meal Planning
- Fitness For Adults With Emotional Disorders (Bulimia/ Bi-Polar Disorder)
- Functional Senior Fitness

I use many different styles of training to foster the desired changes my clients are looking for. Being focused on the individual goal is essential in training and learning my client's needs is paramount. I strive in building strong, honest relations with my clients to ensure crystal clear communication and understanding of the role of professional and client.

Cheryl Harris
Wellness, Fitness & Lifestyle Expert
profoundtouch@yahoo.com
www.profoundtouch.com/contact-us/

Rodney Clark, MBA
CEO, IBT Fitness
Certified Personal Trainer
Independent Herbalife Distributor

Insanebodytrain Fitness (IBT) is located in Savannah, GA it serves the aforementioned, Richmond Hill, Hinesville, and Effingham County. Areas of expertise include personal training, group training, Tabata training, athlete development and fitness camps. Herbalife nutrition product packages are also marketed by this company focusing on weight management, targeted nutrition, athlete nutrition with Herbalife 24 series products. The company has the capability to service clients via online, Skype, and other long distance methods available through current technology servicing clients in New Jersey, Florida, North Carolina, and locally.

- For IBT Fitness workout plans or nutrition options contact us at insanebodytrain@gmail.com.
- For Herbalife products and services visit my website www. goherbalife.com/insanebodytrain.

Workout Videos

There are a number of videos you can use to work out from the comfort of your own home. You can buy videos you see on TV, online, or from stores. Some examples of well-vetted video programs include P90x, T25, Insanity, Taebo, Complete Pregnancy Fitness with Erin O'brien, Dance Off the Inches, Zumba and Total Body Pilates. You could also work out to videos on YouTube, which is free and has a lot of variety. If you don't know where to start, I will give you some YouTube workouts that I have been doing for a couple of years that I love.

Tiffany Rothe has a YouTube channel called TiffanyRothe Workouts. Tiffany Rothe Workouts are fun and effective 10 minute routines that you can mix and match to help you lose body fat, tighten your butt, shrink your waist and firm your back and arms. If you subscribe, you can also be the first to get new workouts! Not only have I seen great changes with my body doing Tiffany Rothe Workouts, but so have many other women.

"Hard work ALWAYS Pays Off!" Karina F

Here are a few of her workouts: Fabulous Fat Burning Workout, Waist Shrinking Tummy Tightening Workout and Sexy Upper Body Workout. My personal favorite is the 10 min Booty Shaking

Waist Workout.

There are other channels that you can also use for your workouts: FitnessBlender is for men and women. This channel provides you with free full-length workouts that include bodyweight workouts, HIIT (High Intensity Interval Training), strength training, cardio, Pilates, kettlebell, yoga, circuit training, low impact, stretching, and more. It contains workout videos for literally every fitness level, from very beginner to incredibly advanced.

"Healthy Lifestyle always a beginning never ending."
Ruby P.

The BeFit Channel provides you with high-quality workouts on Lionsgate BeFit that are sure to keep you looking and feeling your best. Re-shape your body, burn fat, and sculpt lean muscle as you work out with top fitness trainers like Jillian Michaels, Denise Austin, Jane Fonda, Billy Blanks Jr., Scott Herman, Samantha Clayton, Garrett Amerine, Rainbeau Mars, Bryan Tanaka, Sadie Nardini, Dr. Deepak Chopra, Envy Girls, Kym Johnson, Tara Stiles, and many more. Slim your waistline and tone your arms, legs, abs, chest and butt right from your living room for free.

Cassey Ho offers a lively and lighthearted pop culture approach to yoga and fitness instruction, ideal for a younger audience. Her work outs can be found on Blogilates.

SparkPeople Videos has playlists ready to go for pregnancy workouts, swimsuit bootcamps, healthy cooking classes and more.

Yogasync.TV boasts a huge library of guided yoga lessons that, if you can spare 20 minutes three times a week, will help you learn the ancient art in your own home.

Diet.com Video Diet.com has over 500 videos (with over 103,000,000 views) that cover all aspects of exercise, weight loss, nutrition and healthy eating.

"Humans are like pebbles. No two of us are the same. What works for one person may not necessarily work for you. But once you find what works for you stick to it with determination and you can achieve anything you put your mind to." Kiran K.

Scott Herman Fitness. Scott Herman's channel offers new routines and exercises every week with questions and answers, contests and vlogs (video blogs).

Sculpt Your Abs and Burn Fat Jillian Michaels' Six-Pack Abs Workout is 30 minutes of fat-burning cardio that sculpts the abs as well as the arms and legs. The best part? There's instruction for beginners and more advanced exercisers so you can continue to push yourself throughout the full six weeks.

Get Intense With a Bootcamp. Add boot camp workouts to your routine with the BCx Bootcamp videos that include jumps, kicks, pushups and everything in between. Ranging from 4-15 minutes, you can rev up your metabolism with a quickie in the morning or mix and match for a longer workout. Plus, fitness trainer Steve Pfiester words of encouragement will help you charge through.

Turbulence Training was created by Craig Ballantyne. His training is designed for peak fat loss and he offers some great full-length hardcore workouts on his channel. I prefer his routines to some of the other more popular "hardcore" workout channels out there because Ballantyne really knows his stuff and explains the "how" and "why" behind his exercise selection well, which is really important for safety when it comes to high intensity routines. If you like to work hard and push yourself to your limits, then check out his channel!

Brittany MissFitBrit Ramsey. Learn total body conditioning for everyday use to become fit, healthy and increase your motivation, confidence, and encouragement as you view new techniques for functional movement!! If you are getting sick of knee aches and pains in your lower back or other extremities then MissFitBritt is here to help you!! Get Fit with MissFitBritt and become a member of the Rock Hard Boot Camps for all fitness levels, come train with MissFitBritt for Personal Training packages and get MissFitBritt to come speak to your company, or organization as she is also a Motivational Speaker as it relates to Health n Wellness of Life!!

"Building a strong core is the beginning of building a stronger you." Stephanie M.

TONIC focuses on Yoga moves for just about anything and other workout videos. The length of the videos range from 10 minutes to even under a minute.

Nicole Chaplin focuses on intense and targeted workouts. Her videos are great for those who want to intensify their workouts. She focuses on everything from partner workouts to bootcamps. Her videos are under three minutes. You can find her on Instagram.

Sixpack Shortcuts focuses on abs with trainer Mike Chang. He focuses on all things abs: from losing belly fat to gaining muscle to building a stronger core. His videos usually are 15 minute in length

You no longer have any excuse not to work out. I have given you the option to choose from a number of free work outs, from walking/running to using YouTube videos. You can pay for a trainer or buy videos to do your work outs. And of course, you can also join a gym, but if you do this, please, please, buy books or magazines that show you what exercises to do and the correct form to use when performing them. I don't want you to hurt yourself while working out. Also, please, listen to your body. This means, if you are too exhausted (not just lazy!) please rest. If you have an injury, please take care of your injury before exercising that area again. As you can see I did not say, don't exercise at all, unless you have to or your doctor has told you to stop. I have given you many ways to get start, pick one and get started tomorrow. Now, what did you say your excuse was again?

———————

" "If you can USE YOUR ENERY to complain, you can use your energy to CHANGE." Sherwood G

———————

Tracking Your Progress

The Scale

There are a number of ways to track your progress along your healthy lifestyle journey. One of my least favorite ways to track progress is by stepping on the scale. We have become so addicted to weighing ourselves on the scale that it does more harm than good. We are always looking to get back to that "low weight", not realizing that when we start working out, eating healthfully and losing body fat, we are going to look like we weigh less than what the scale reads.

A lot of people say, "Muscle weighs less than fat." Untrue: Five pounds of muscle is the same as five pounds of fat. However, five pounds of muscle takes up less room than five pounds of fat. This explains why a 150 pound woman who exercises and eats healthfully looks smaller than a woman who weighs the same but who doesn't live a healthy life style. If you are exercising and eating healthfully then stop concentrating so much on the scale, unless you like being frustrated. I will give you another example. Let's say your goal weight is 140 pounds. The last time you weighed 140 pounds, you wore a size 8. As you exercise and begin to eat healthfully, the number on the scale reads 145 but you wear a size 6. Because you are so stuck on the number on the scale you don't realize that you are actually smaller than you were when you wore a size 8.

"If you just don't stop, it's inevitable that y ou'll reach your goals!" Cawanda E.

Do I weigh myself? Yes, I do, but I don't focus on that number. I use the scale to make sure I don't get under a certain number.

If you are going to weigh yourself, do it first thing in the morning after using the bathroom. This gives your body time to digest the food from the day before and also to eliminate waste. You don't want to weigh yourself throughout the day because our weight can fluctuate between 3-5 pounds on any given day.

I will also suggest if you want to weigh yourself, to limit your weigh ins to once a month. Weighing yourself every day is unnecessary and can become an addiction that can turn into frustration and stress (which builds up cortisol fat in the body and this fat is stored or moved to your abdomen.) Eliminating this source of stress will help with your weight loss and the number on the scale.

Your Measurements

Another way to track your progress is by taking your measurements once a month. Like your weight, you shouldn't take your measurements daily. You are not going to see big change daily. Below is a diagram of where and how you should take your measurements. I have also provided you with a measurement tracking sheet, located in the appendix.

*"Open your mind & heart up to change
and change will find you!" Aretha M.*

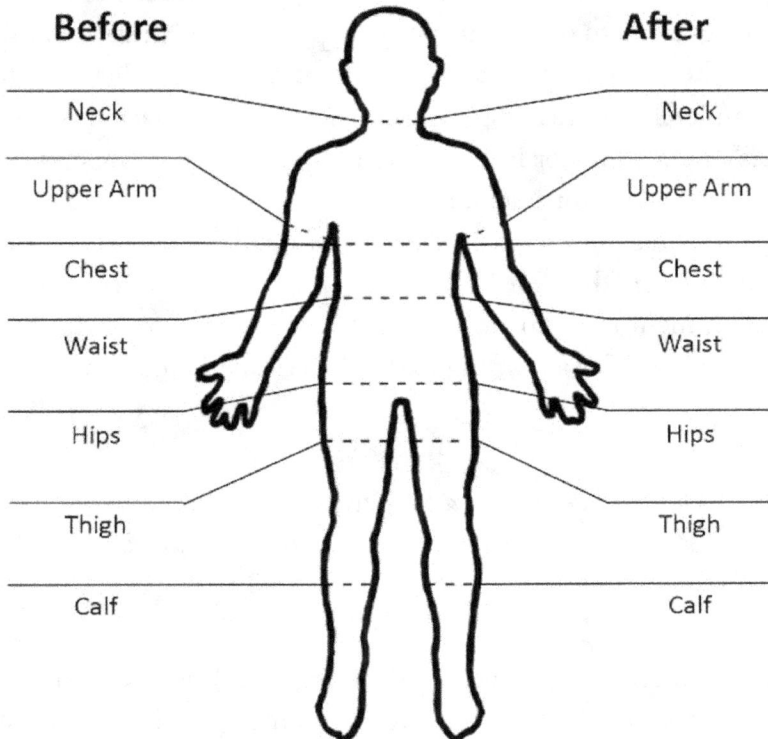

Before   **After**

Neck   Neck

Upper Arm   Upper Arm

Chest   Chest

Waist   Waist

Hips   Hips

Thigh   Thigh

Calf   Calf

Body Fat Tests

You can also track your progress by keeping track of your body fat. This can be done several ways. Before getting into a discussion of tracking your body fat, I want to mention BMI, or Body Mass Index. A lot of doctors use your BMI to determine if you are obese. Your BMI is simply a ratio of weight (in kilograms) divided by height (in meters) squared and **does not** take into account what your body is actually made of, specifically: lean body mass like muscle, bone and water versus fat.

The three methods of measuring body fat I am going to discuss are: underwater weighing (hydrostatic weighing) test, Skinfold caliper test and BOD POD® test. An underwater weighing test determines body density by measuring the weight of the body outside the water, the weight of the body underwater after exhaling completely, and the density of the water. The resulting body density is then put into an equation to determine body fat percentage. There are limitations to the accuracy of this test. Many people have difficulty exhaling completely before being submerged, and a person can hold up to 4 liters of gas in his or her system at any given time. Bone mineral density also varies considerably from person to person (larger-boned people may have more air in their bones, which can affect density measurements). This test is fairly expensive and requires considerable equipment to perform. The measurement of error of this test is approximately 2.7% according to the American Council on Exercise.

"Our lives begin to end the day we become silent about things that matter most to our lives." Eman A.

The skinfold caliper test is generally the least expensive and mostly widely available. It involves pinching specific areas of skin (and fat) throughout the body and converting the results into an estimate to body fat percentage. While it does provide regional body fat assessment, it does not measure deep belly fat, which is very important in terms of health. There is considerable variability in general as to where people carry extra fat, and it is more difficult to get accurate measurements in the extremely obese. In addition, the test is very dependent on the person performing the test and the quality of the calipers used. In the hands of a qualified person, a skinfold caliper test can provide a good relative measure of body fat percentage.

The third test I'll discuss is the BOD POD®. BOD POD® technology is fundamentally the same as underwater (hydrostatic) weighing, but uses air instead of water. The BOD POD® measures the volume of air a person's body displaces while sitting inside a comfortable chamber, rather than measuring how much water his or her body displaces when dunked in a tank. By using air instead of water, the BOD POD® offers a fast, safe, and easy-to-use tool for measuring body composition, without sacrificing accuracy.

Since it is based on the same whole-body measurement principle as hydrostatic weighing, the BOD POD® first measures the subject's mass and volume. From these measurements, whole-body density is determined. Using this data, body fat and lean mass can then be calculated.

"Plan to do and do as you plan. "Phillip B. IFBB Pro

Research studies at major universities have established the outstanding accuracy, safety and speed of the BOD POD®. Before the BOD POD®, the most accepted method for measuring body fat percentage was underwater weighing. When comparing the two methods, the BOD POD® and underwater weighing often produce identical results. Many top scientists consider the BOD POD® to be even more accurate than underwater weighing because testing with the BOD POD® is so easy. The general error range of the BOD POD® is 1-2% (the same as hydrostatic weighing).

I have used two of the three tests I discussed. I have a skinfold caliper at home I use once a month. This is just to help me determine if my body fat has gone up or if it has gone down. I test the area 3 times to make sure I get the same number. Once a year I will have the BOD POD® test done. Before having the BOD POD® test done, I will use the skinfold caliper to determine how accurate the skinfold test is compared to the BOD POD® test.

Clothing

One of the simplest ways to track your progress is by monitoring how your clothes are fitting. Everyone loves when their clothes begin to fit loose; this means, what you are doing is working. Then again, once your clothes begin to get *too* big, it can be hard for you to tell if you've made further progress because you are so used to wearing loose clothes. I've been guilty of wearing loose clothes far longer than I should, waiting to buy new clothes until I reached a certain look. The real danger is wearing pants so loose that they surprise you by falling down in public! Try to avoid this.

My suggestion is to buy clothes from a resale or thrift store until you reach the size you want to be in. You will save money in the long run. Why buy new clothes when in a month or less you will no longer be able to wear them?

"Ready, set, fit! Paulina So

You may want to try another method, too, when it comes to tracking your progress with your clothes. All of us have something in our closet that is a little small or too tight for us to wear. Put on that skirt, jacket, or pair of jeans and take a picture of how you look with nothing covering the top of the clothing. (I know your stomach is going to be showing but that is okay .If you don't like what you see, this will be great motivation.) Take a front and a side picture of yourself. In one month, after exercising and eating healthfully for one month, take a new picture with the same clothing on and notice the difference.

Monthly Pictures

My favorite way to track my progress is by taking monthly pictures. Every four weeks, not only do I take pictures, but I also take my measurements. You may not see a difference at first, but as the months go by, you will be able to see yourself getting smaller and smaller. I also like to take monthly pictures because at the end of the year I have tracked my entire progress and can share those with others.

When taking your pictures, take them in something tight. Wear something tight because you will be able to see your body change more easily than in loose clothes.

"Regardless of what you currently look like, love yourself unconditionally while you are traveling down the fitness road." Otisa J.

How Long will it Take to See a Difference?

Everyone's body is different, so there's not a one-size-fits-all answer to how long it will take to see changes in your body when you start working out. It also depends largely on the kind of workouts you're doing, and what your lifestyle is like. Working out once every couple of weeks is not going to give you much in the way of noticeable changes. You might feel good once you've done it, but you won't lose any weight, gain any muscle definition or improve your cardiovascular health. Including three to five workouts a week can help you see changes in your weight, health and your body's appearance within the first month or two of starting training.

Your body is unlikely to respond noticeably to gentle exercise—it needs to be tough. Not so tough that you're in pain or unable to move by the end of it, but enough that you are worn out and don't feel capable of doing any more. Ensuring your workouts are demanding will help you to see results more quickly than if you are just doing easy, but long, workouts.

When setting your goals for the month, be realistic, please. Losing 30 pounds in one month is unrealistic. You should lose about 1-2 pounds a week on average. You did not put the weight on overnight, which means it isn't going to come off overnight. It will come off faster than you put it on and as long as you are being consistent, focused, and committed to your workouts and eating well you will see progress. Remember, slow progress is better than no progress at all.

———◦◉◦———

"The ATTITUDE of one can affect so man. The FAITH of one can inspire the world." Phillip B. IFBB Pro

———◦◉◦———

Below are the pictures I took over one year, and I definitely was happy I did.

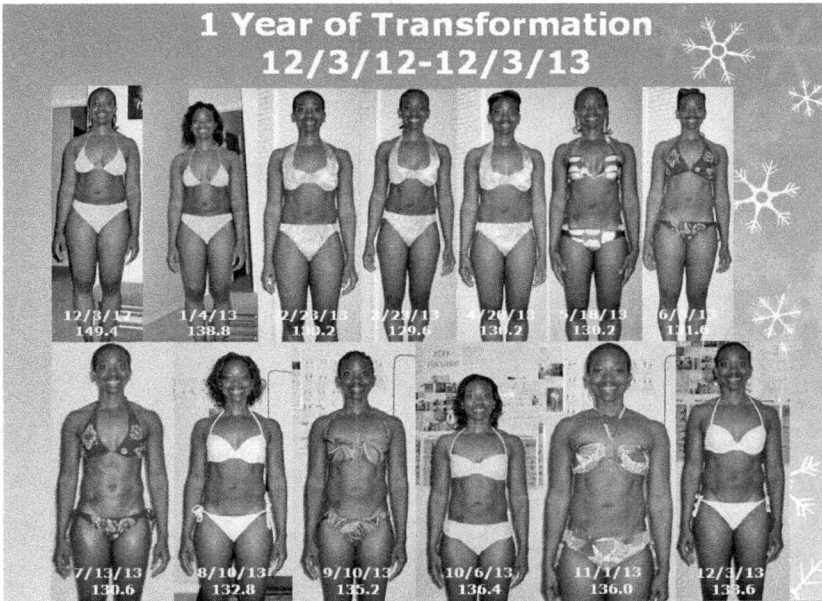

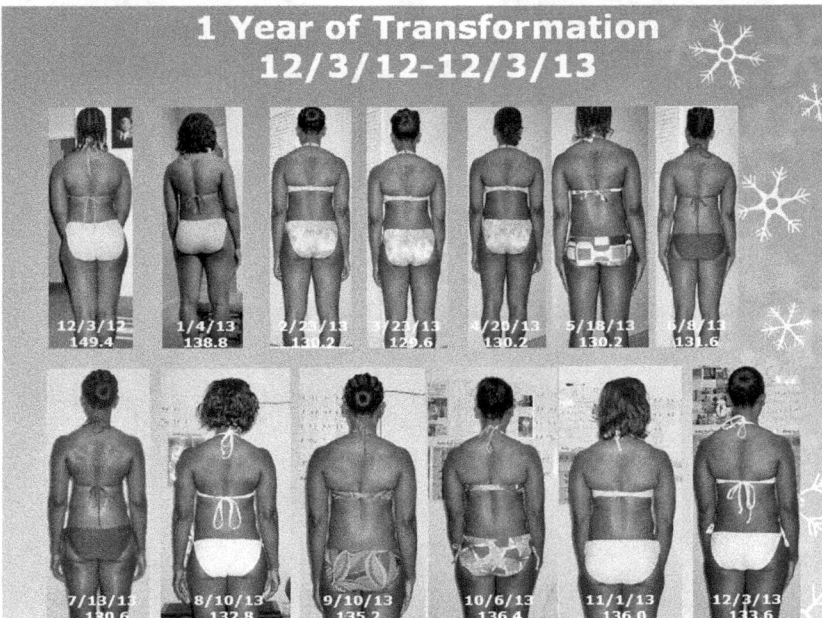

*"The days I don't want to go are the days I go the hardest
I will not be defeated by my enemy which is my inner
me." Cassive C. Esq.*

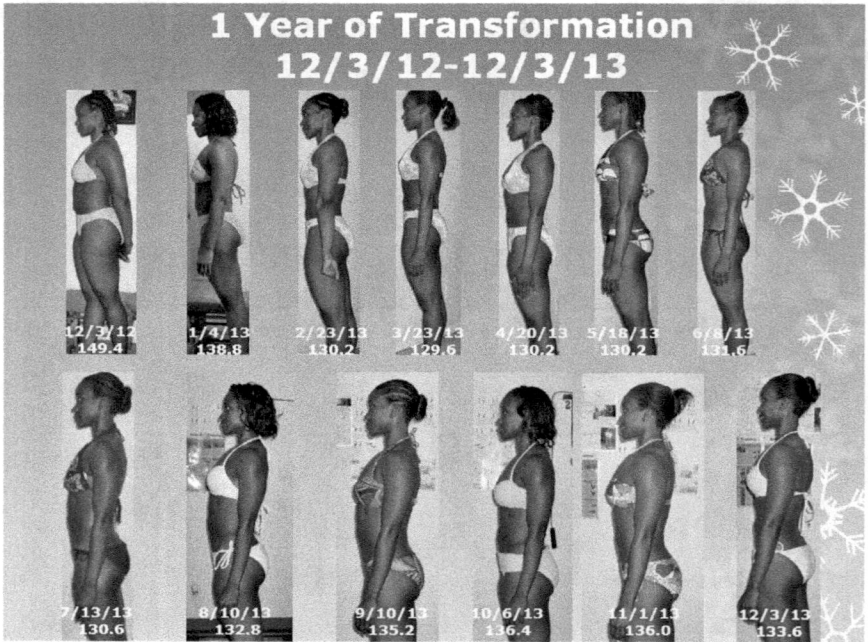

"The magic word is: consistency. Get up, fall down, get up. Just continue every day a little bit. Don't give up!"
Heike F.

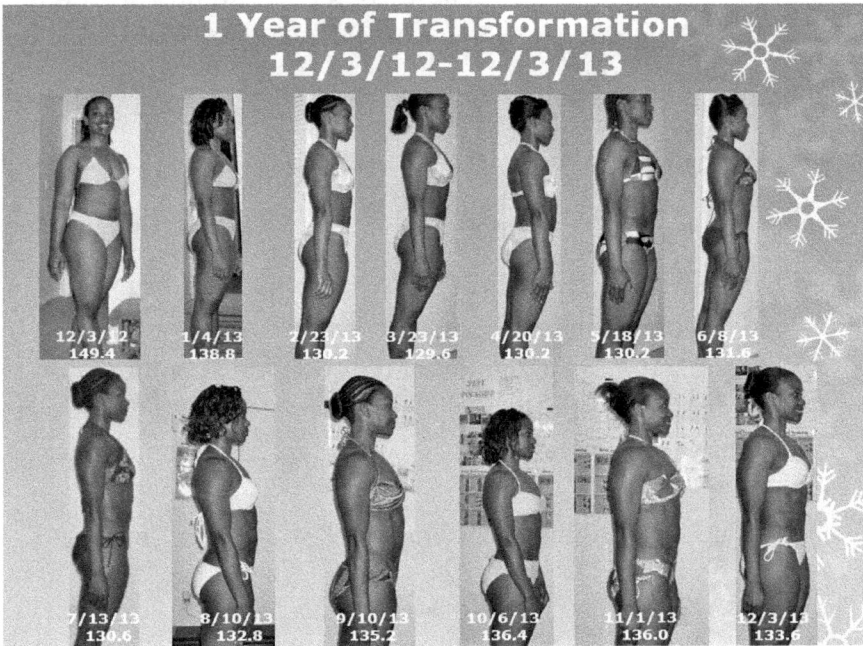

1 Year of Transformation
12/3/12-12/3/13

Chapter 7
Sample Workouts

B efore starting any new exercises, or a conditioning or workout program, consult your physician. The workouts in this chapter are suggested workouts.

- Women should do 3 sets of 12-15 reps.
- Men should do 3 sets of 8-10 reps

What are "reps"? Reps (short for "repetitions") are the number of times you perform an exercise, or lift a weight.

What is a set? A set is a group of reps performed without rest. If you perform 10 reps of dumbbell curls without resting, this is considered a set. It is often best to rest about 90 to 120 seconds between each set.

Warm up for 5-10 minutes before each workout.

———◉———

*"The moments you feel things are pulling you back,
you're really just getting a small tug that will propel you
forward in a burst of energy." Daphna S.*

———◉———

Warning:

The following exercises should never be performed if they cause irritation to any part of your body while they are being performed! As each exercise is different, always consult your doctor before performing any of these exercises to determine what exercises, if any, are right for you. If you have any discomfort after performing any of these exercises, discontinue immediately and consult a doctor to properly assess your situation. If you have any knee or back injuries, avoid these exercises due to the impact involved. Also, make certain when doing any jumping exercise that your landings are controlled and that you land with your two feet straight (toes touching the floor first when jumping). The wrong landing can result in a sprained ligament.

"The temple needs substance not bulk!!!" Babette D.

Sample Week Workout

MONDAY:
Quads
Squats

1. Place feet about shoulder-width apart.
2. Point your feet slightly outward, not straight ahead.
3. Never let your knees extend beyond your toes.
4. Look straight ahead. Bend at your knees as if you were going to sit back in a chair, keeping your heels on the floor.
5. Pull in your abs, and keep your lower back in a near neutral position (a slightly arched back might be unavoidable).
6. Tighten your whole body when you perform the squat.
7. Lower yourself. In a controlled manner slowly lower yourself down and back so that your upper legs are nearly parallel with the floor. Keep the upper body tight at all times.
8. Repeat for the recommended amount of repetitions.

———◈———

"Time to rebuild or finally create the world you've always wanted. You are more powerful than you imagine. STOP DOUBTING & START DOING."
Phillip B. IFBB Pro

———◈———

Smith Machine

1. Set the bar on the height that best matches your height. Once the correct height is chosen and the bar is loaded, step under the bar and place the back of your shoulders (slightly below the neck) across it.
2. Hold on to the bar using both arms at each side (palms facing forward), unlock it and lift it off the rack by first pushing with your legs and at the same time straightening your torso.
3. Position your legs using a shoulder width medium stance with the toes slightly pointed out. Keep your head up at all times and your back straight.
4. Begin to squat by bending your knees, keeping your back straight and head up. Squat down until your legs are parallel or 90 degrees (parallel to the floor) Inhale as you squat down. You knees should never go past your toes. (If you knees go past your toes you are putting unnecessary pressure or stress on your knees).
5. Begin to stand up as you breathe out to the starting position.
6. Repeat for the recommended amount of repetitions.

———◆———

"Trust the process because it works." Zhivi W.

———◆———

Walking lunges

These can also be performed with dumbbells.

1. Stand tall with good posture, with your hands on your hips
2. Step far forward with one leg while simultaneously lifting up onto the ball of the back foot.
3. While allowing your chest to remain high in the air and keeping your shoulders back, bend the knees and drop your hips downwards straight to the ground. Your back knee should not touch the floor and your front knee shouldn't go over your toe. Ensure that the back knee does not touch the floor and that the front knee does not move too far forward.
4. Press up with your front leg and bring the back foot forward.
5. Take another step forward with the opposite leg and repeat the lunge.

"Unless you limit what you are capable of doing, there are no limits to what you are able to achieve fitness wise. Don't let your negative thinking hold you back." Otisa J

Step ups

This can be performed using a bench or a stable chair

1. Begin by standing in front of the bench or chair facing forward.
2. Place right foot in the middle of the bench or step and step up as you balance your body for 1-2 seconds on the right leg.
3. Your left leg should be behind your body to help stabilize your weight as it is shifting.
4. Step down with your left leg first and continue on down with your right.
5. Try for 2 sets of 10-12 repetitions for each leg.
6. To make this exercise more difficult, add dumbbells.

Jumping squats

1. Stand with your feet shoulder-width apart and your head up and back straight.
2. Keeping your back straight and chest up do a regular squat. As you squat down, inhale until your upper thighs are parallel or lower to the floor, then engage your core and jump up as high as you can.
3. When you land, lower your body back into the squat position to complete one rep. Land as quietly as possible, which requires control.
4. Do two to three sets of 10 reps.
5. To make this exercise more difficult, add dumbbells.

"We hide our gifts and talents in excuses that distract us from our purpose." Dr. Verletta S.

Using the Leg Press Machine

1. Sit down on the machine and place your legs on the platform directly in front of you with your feet shoulder width apart.

2. Lower the safety bars holding the weighted platform in place and press the platform all the way up until your legs are fully extended in front of you without locking your knees. (Leave the safety bars on for increased safety.) Your torso and the legs should make perfect 90-degree angle.

3. Carefully place your toes and balls of your feet on the lower portion of the platform with the heels extending off. Toes should be facing forward, outwards or inwards (Be careful as you place your feet on the bottom part of the platform because your feet could slip if the safety bars are not locked and you could suffer a serious injury.)

4. Press on the platform by raising your heels as you breathe out by extending your ankles as high as possible and flexing your calf. Don't lock your knees. Hold the contracted position by a second before you start to go back down.

5. Go back slowly to the starting position as you breathe in by lowering your heels as you bend the ankles until calves are stretched.

Inner Thigh

Pilates Inner-Thigh Leg Lifts

1. Lying on your side, lengthen your bottom leg and cross your top leg over it. Rest either your knee or foot on the floor. Prop your head up with your hand, or rest your head on your arm.
2. As you exhale, lift your bottom leg up, and inhale as you lower it back down. Your torso should stay still while you do this

---

"We are like tea bags we don't know our own strength until we're in hot water." Eman A.

Outer Thigh

Fire hydrants – Bent Knee

1. Place your body on an all-fours position. Elbows should be slightly bent.
2. Back should be parallel to the ground, not arched or swayed downward.
3. Keeping the kneeling position raise left leg out to the side, parallel to the ground. Maintain for a second and slowly return to the initial position.
4. Repeat movement with same leg until set is finished. Repeat the exercise using the right leg.

Fire hydrants – Straight leg

1. Place your body on an all-fours position. Elbows should be slightly bent.
2. Back should be parallel to the ground, not arched or swayed downward.
3. Keeping the kneeling position raise left leg out to the side, parallel to the ground. Maintain for a second and slowly return to the initial position.
4. Repeat movement with same leg until set is finished. Repeat the exercise using the right leg.

"We often tell our life stories as if we were victims instead of survivors. You are a survivor." Dr. Verletta S.

Calves
Calf raise

You will need a chair or a wall when performing this exercise at home.

1. Stand up straight, grasping a chair or wall for balance.
2. Position your feet hip-width apart.
3. Slowly raise your heels until you're on your tiptoes. Balance your body weight on the balls of your feet.
4. Pause for a minute, and then slowly lower yourself.

To make this exercise more difficult, use one leg at a time.

———◦———

"When the thought appears: I can't - have you tried it today? Is it true? Go and find out by doing! You can!"
Heike F.

———◦———

TUESDAY:
Chest/Back
Dumbbell bench press (if you don't have a bench you will lay on the floor)

1. Sit down on bench/floor with dumbbells in your hands. If you are sitting on the floor bend your knees at a 90 degree angle.
2. Lift the weights to your shoulder and lie back.
3. Position dumbbells to sides of chest with bent arm under each dumbbell.
4. Press dumbbells up with elbows to sides until arms are extended.
5. Lower weight to sides of upper chest until slight stretch is felt in chest or shoulder (you will feel this stretch if lying on a bench).

———◦———

"Being healthy and fit isn't a fad that comes and goes, it's a lifestyle" Vincent F.

———◦———

Dumbbell flys

1. Sit down on bench/floor with dumbbells in your hands. If you are sitting on the floor bend your knees at a 90 degree angle.
2. Lie back on the bench/floor, extend your arms out, holding the dumbbells above your body your palms facing each other. The dumbbells should not be touching. If on a bench, keep your feet planted on the floor for balance. Bend your arms slightly. This is your starting position.
3. Slowly lower the dumbbells out to your sides, keeping your arms slightly bent.
4. Once the dumbbells get about level with your chest, squeeze the chest muscles and raise the dumbbells back up.
5. Without letting the dumbbells touch, slowly lower them again.

———

"You are a product of your unwillingness to do something about them." Tanisha B.

———

Pushups

Don't do pushups if you suffer from a neck or shoulder injury. Don't let your back sag down or your hips rise up.

You can also do pushups on your knees.

1. Begin on your hands and knees with your hands underneath your shoulders but slightly wider than your shoulders.
2. Come onto the balls of your feet and the heels of your hands,

and then walk the feet back until you're in the plank position.

3. Keep your hips lifted to avoid the lower back bowing so the belly sags towards the ground.

4. Begin to bend your elbows, lowering your body in one solid piece down towards the floor. Your elbows will bend out to the side, not behind you.

5. Keep your abdominal and leg muscles engaged throughout the entire movement. Your head should stay in line with your spine, not droop.

6. Lower yourself down until your chest is about an inch or two from the ground and then slowly push yourself back up to the starting position.

"You are defined by what you believe. Let the weak say I am strong. Attitude is everything." Phillip B. IFBB Pro

---

Pull-ups

If doing pull ups in the gym, you can use the assisted pull-ups machine. If you would like to do these at home you will need to buy a pull-up doorway bar. Use a chair at home to assist you if you are unable to do them with no assistance.

1. Stand below pull-up bar and grasp it with wide overhand grip. Hang on bar.

2. Bend your knees and cross your lower legs.

3. Pull your body up until your upper chest reaches the bar. Look up and keep chest up, leading toward the bar.

4. Return with same speed. Keep the arms very slightly bent at

the bottom of the motion to maintain the muscular activity. Simultaneously let your shoulders are pulled up by the bodyweight.

———◆———

"You have the power to turn your fitness dream into a fitness reality. Paulina S.

———◆———

Bent over dumbbell rows

These can also be done at home by using a chair.

1. Place a dumbbell on the floor next to the bench/chair.
2. Kneel over side of bench/chair by placing knee and hand of supporting arm on bench/chair.
3. Position foot of opposite leg slightly back to side.
4. Grab the dumbbell from floor. The dumbbell should be on the same side with the foot that is on the floor.
5. Pull dumbbell to up to side until it makes contact with ribs or until upper arm is just beyond horizontal.
6. Return until arm is extended and shoulder is stretched downward.

Reverse flys

1. Grab dumbbells in hands.
2. Place feet shoulder wide apart, bend knees and hips to lean forward. Keep back straight.
3. Hold dumbbells below chest and keep arms slightly flexed.
4. Raise arms to sides until elbows are slightly higher than shoulders.

WHO NEEDS A GYM?

5. Keep upper arms perpendicular to body and elbows pointing up.

Superman

1. Lie straight and face down on the floor or exercise mat. Your arms should be fully extended in front of you.
2. Raise your arms, legs, and chest off of the floor at the same time and hold this contraction for 2 seconds.
3. Squeeze your lower back and exhale during this movement. When holding the contracted position, you should look like superman when he is flying.
4. Slowly begin to lower your arms, legs and chest back down to the starting position while inhaling.

Cardio: 30–45 minutes

"You have to love where you are first, that you can appreciate where you want to go." Dennis R.

WEDNESDAY:
Abs
Bicycle crunch

1. Lie flat on the floor or mat, with your lower back pressed to the ground and contract your stomach muscles.
2. Place your hands behind your head and bring your legs up with your knees at a 90 degree angle.
3. With your hands gently holding your head, elbows pointed to the sides, straighten your left knee while keeping your right knee bent.
4. Bring your left elbow toward your right knee. Alternately touching your elbows to the opposite knees as you twist back and forth.
5. Breathe evenly throughout the exercise.
6. Knee in
7. Sit on the floor (or on the edge of a chair or bench) with your legs extended in front of you and your hands holding on to the sides for support.
8. Keeping your knees together, pull your knees in towards your chest until you can go no farther.
9. Keeping the tension on your lower ab muscles, return to the start position.

"You are capable of so much more than you think. So, learn to love the process, the off days, the bad days because there will come a time where you realize that what you thought was impossible is now possible. Dr. Harriet D. IFBB Bikini Pro

Plank

1. Lay face down on the floor/mat.
2. Place your forearms on the floor. Your arms are bent directly below your shoulders. Your weight is being supported by your toes and your forearms.
3. Keep your body straight at all times, and hold this position as long as possible.

"Finding beads of pearls in life enriches ones virtues beyond personal belief." Pamela R.

Twisting crunch

1. Lie on your back with your feet on the floor and your knees at a 90 degree angle. Place your hands behind your head.
2. Exhale as you lift your shoulder blades off the floor.
3. When you get half way up, start to rotate your body so that your left elbow moves towards your right knee.
4. Hold at the top for 1 second and slowly lower to the starting position.
5. Complete one set with your left elbow then with the right elbow.

SAMPLE WORKOUTS

Side planks

1. Lie on your side on a mat/floor.
2. Place your left forearm on mat/floor under shoulder perpendicular to body.
3. Place upper leg directly on top of lower leg and straighten knees and hips.
4. Raise body upward by straightening waist so body is ridged. Hold as long as you can.
5. Repeat with your right side.

Cardio 45-60 minute cardio

"Greatest cost, what it cost, it's a full commitment that you must be willing to pay" Darius "Buff" M.

THURSDAY:
Bicep/Triceps

For biceps and triceps you can use dumbbell weights, cans, water bottles filled with dirt, sand or water.

Standing bicep curls

1. Stand up straight holding a dumbbell in each hand.
2. Your arms should be straight in front of you with your palms facing forward.
3. Keep your back straight, shoulders back and tighten your stomach muscles.
4. At the same time, curl the dumbbells up until shoulder height, keeping your elbows next to your side.
5. Pause briefly at the top and squeeze your bicep muscles
6. Slowly lower back to the start position

Standing hammer curls

1. Stand up straight holding a dumbbell in each hand.
2. Your arms should be straight next to your sides with your palms facing inward (facing your thighs).
3. Keep your back straight, shoulders back and tighten your stomach muscles.
4. At the same time, curl the dumbbells up until shoulder height, keeping your elbows next to your side.
5. Pause briefly at the top and squeeze your bicep muscles.
6. Slowly lower back to the start position.

"Your Voice Is The Only Truth" Karen C.

Seated concentration curls

1. Grab a dumbbell.
2. Sit on a bench or chair with feet a little more than should width a part and the dumbbell on the floor between your feet.
3. Grab the dumbbell in your right hand and place back of your right upper arm to your right inner thigh.
4. Lean into your right leg to raise your right elbow slightly.
5. Raise the dumbbell to your right front of shoulder.
6. Lower the dumbbell until your right arm is fully extended.
7. Complete one set.
8. Repeat using your left arm.

Dumbbell kick backs

1. Place a dumbbell on the left hand side of a bench or chair.
2. Stand on the left side of the bench or chair with your right knee and right hand on the bench or chair.
3. Pick up the dumbbell with your left hand. Keep your back straight, bend over and look forward.
4. Your left elbow should be close to your torso and bent, forming a 90 degree angle with your arm.
5. Moving only at the elbow, raise the dumbbell behind you until your arm is fully extended.
6. Complete one set.
7. Repeat using your right arm.

Standing 1 arm tricep extension

1. Stand up straight with a dumbbell held in your left hand.
2. Your feet should be about shoulder width apart from each other.
3. Fully extend your left arm with the dumbbell over your head. The dumbbell should be above your head.
4. Keeping your upper left arm close to your head (elbows in) and perpendicular to the floor, lower the dumbbell behind your head until your forearm touch your bicep. Your left arm should remain stationary and only the forearm should move.
5. Breathe in as you perform this step.
6. Raise the dumbbell and breathe out.
7. Complete one set.
8. Repeat using your right arm.

———◈———

"You have to want success, someone can't hand it to you."
Dennis R.

———◈———

Dips

For this exercise you can use a chair, bench or the floor.
1. Place your hands beside you on the bench/chair/floor with your feet placed out in front of you.
2. Keeping your back straight and your tailbone close to the bench/chair (if you are using the floor, you will not keep your back straight) lower yourself until your arms are at a 90 degree.
3. Raise yourself back up by fully extending your arms and contracting your triceps muscles.

Cardio: 30 minutes

FRIDAY:
Shoulders/Butt
Dumbbell shoulder press

1. While holding a dumbbell in each hand, sit on a military press, utility bench or chair that has back support.
2. Raise the dumbbells to shoulder so that your arms are 90 degrees.
3. Make sure to rotate your wrists so that your palms are facing forward.
4. Exhale and push the dumbbells upward until they touch at the top.
5. After a brief pause at the top contracted position, slowly lower the weights back down to 90 degrees.

Standing lateral raises

1. Stand up straight with a dumbbell in each hand by your side at arm's length with the palms of the hand facing you.
2. As you continue to stand straight, don't swing; lift the dumbbells to your side with a slight bend on the elbow and the hands slightly tilted forward as if pouring water in a glass.
3. Bring your arms up unit they are parallel to the floor.
4. Exhale as you bring your arms up.
5. Pause for a second at the top.
6. Lower the dumbbells back down slowly to your sides.

———————

""Walk in your GREATNESS & share it with the WORLD. BE AWESOME!!!" Phillip B.

———————

Front dumbbell raises

1. Stand up straight with a dumbbell in each hand and the dumbbells on your thighs at arm's length with the palms of the hand facing your thighs.
2. While standing with a straight back, no swinging; lift the left dumbbells to the front with a slight bend on the elbow and the palms of the hands always facing down.
3. Bring your arms up until your arms are slightly above parallel to the floor.
4. Breach out and pause for a second at the top. Inhale after the second pause.
5. Lower the dumbbell down slowly, keeping your arms and back straight.

Upright rows

1. Stand up straight with a dumbbell in each hand and the dumbbells on your thighs at arm's length with the palms of the hand facing your thighs.
2. Pull dumbbells up to your shoulder with elbows leading out to sides.
3. Allow wrists to flex as dumbbells rise upward.

———◉———

*"Too often we underestimate the power of our mindset.
Remember to keep it positive!" Dr. Harriet D IFBB Bikini Pro.*

———◉———

Donkey kicks

1. Get on your hands and knees, with your wrists under your shoulders and knees under your hips.
2. Drawing your abs in, lift your left leg parallel to the floor, with knee bent, foot flexed.
3. Slowly kick leg in the air.
4. Fully extend leg up as high as you can.
5. Lower the leg until the knee is just below parallel to the floor.

———◉———

*"**Don't** believe me...just watch Wont
HE do it....yes HE will." Michelle A*

———◉———

Leg abduction

1. Get on your hands and knees, with your wrists under your shoulders and knees under your hips. Elbows should be slightly bent.
2. Your back should be parallel to the ground, not arched or swayed downward.
3. Keeping the kneeling position raise left leg out to the side, parallel to the ground. Maintain for a second and slowly return.
4. Repeat the exercise using the right leg.

Cardio: 30 minutes

Sample Routine, Month 2:

HIIT/Cardio

When doing the HIIT (High Intensity Interval Training) routines, the suggested routine below is for beginners. Intermediate and advanced individuals should do more reps.

MONDAY/WEDNESDAY/FRIDAY
Warm up:
Complete two times
1 minute jump rope
1 minute run in place
1 minute jumping jacks

Group 1

Compete four times with no rest in between. After doing 25 high knees, standing in place go right into 25 jumping jacks.

25 jumping jacks
25 standing squats
25 high knees standing in place

1. Stand in place with your feet hip-width apart.
2. Drive your right knee toward your chest and quickly place it back on the ground.
3. Follow immediately by driving your left knee toward your chest.
4. Continue to alternate knees as quickly as you can.

———◈———

"Instant gratification is a lie, enjoy the journey.
It's more fun that way." Justina G.

———◈———

Group 2

Complete five times with a 30 second rest between sets. After completing your pushups take a 30 second rest and start again from the top.

45 seconds fast jump rope
25 bicycle crunches (left elbow to right knee, right elbow to left knee = 1)
20 pushups (can be done on your knees or feet)

"Just because you are associating yourself with fit people doesn't mean that it will make you fit. Remember you have to consistently put in the hard work with clean eating and working out." Otisa J.

Group 3

Complete four times with a 30 second rest between sets.

8-10 burpees

1. Bend over or squat down and place your hands on the floor in front of you, just outside of your feet.
2. Jump both feet back (or walk your feet back) so that you're now in plank position.
3. Do a push up; your chest should touch the floor. You can also drop to your knees here, which makes the impending push-up easier. (You can also skip doing the push up.)
4. Push up to return to plank position. You can also push up from your knees.
5. Jump your feet back (or walk your feet) in toward the hands.
6. Explosively jump into the air, reaching your arms straight overhead (if you are a beginner, don't jump in the air until you are ready to)
7. Start again.

40 walking lunges (20 each leg)
> To make this exercise more difficult you can use dumbbells.

Warnings:
- Bend your knees 90 degrees for a full range of motion
- Don't step too far, or you will exert pressure on your knee.
- Stop if you experience pain in the knee.
- Don't let your knee go over your toes.

1. Stand with your legs shoulder width apart.
2. Step forward with right leg and lower your body to 90 degrees in both knees.
3. Don't step out too far, and drop into a deep lunge.
4. There should be 2 to 2.5 feet between your feet at this point.
5. Keep your right heel in contact with the ground as you stand back up.
6. Make sure to keep your weight on your heels to maintain balance.
7. Push up, bringing the left leg forward until you are standing straight again.
8. Step forward with the right leg and repeat, walking forward.

"Keep starting over until it becomes habit." Cawanda E.

25 mountain climbers

1. Place hands on floor, slightly wider than shoulder width.
2. Bend one leg forward under your body and extend other leg back.
3. While holding upper body in place, alternate leg positions by pushing hips up while immediately extending forward leg back and pulling rear leg forward under body.
4. This should look like you are running in place.

TUESDAY/THURSDAY
Cardio, 45-60 minutes

"Listen to your body as much as your brain,
work together for the goal." Kenroy G.

Chapter 8
What I Personally Do

How Many Times a Day I Eat

I eat all day long. My husband likes to tease that I am greedy, but I don't mind him saying it, because what I eat all day long are lean proteins, fresh fruits and either raw or steamed vegetables, with nuts for snacks. I eat at least five meals a day, consisting of breakfast, a snack, lunch, another snack and dinner. Some healthy people eat six meals a day, and after dinner they will eat another snack. I am usually asleep by this time so I only eat five meals a day. If you eat on a schedule like this, you will eat every two to three hours. I know this may sound like a lot to eat throughout the day, and you will not be hungry enough, but when you start eating like this your body will get used to this schedule, and every two to three hours you will be hungry. Eating five to six meals a day will provide you with energy, and prevent you from eating unhealthy foods when you're hungry and there is only junk food around to eat.

———◈———

"Mind over matter." Michelle A

———◈———

Here is an example of meals I may eat in one day:

Breakfast: Oatmeal, 4 large egg whites and 1 egg and 2 pieces of uncured turkey bacon
Snack: Fresh fruits with nuts (1 serving of nuts)
Lunch: Brown rice, vegetables and baked fish
Snack: Tuna and brown rice (small portion)
Dinner: Chicken breast and vegetables

At each meal, I also drink green tea made with lemon water (without any type of sweetener). Again this is just an example of what I may eat in one day; there are a number of combinations you can have. You want to make sure you eat the following:

Breakfast: Carb, protein and vegetables (you don't always have to have vegetables)
Snack: Carb and protein or fruit and nuts
Lunch: Carb, protein and vegetables
Snack: Carb and protein or fruit and nuts
Dinner: Protein and vegetables

"Most of life is about showing up." Dr. Verletta S.

What I am going to tell you now, some people will agree with and some will disagree with it. You will need to determine what works best for you. There are different ways you can do this. Every week I give myself a "free" day to eat whatever I want all day long. If you decide to follow this practice, PLEASE don't get on the scale the day after you have your free day. I can guarantee that you will have gained weight. If you have been eating healthy food all week and you eat unhealthy foods on one day, all the sodium, water retention, sugar, and whatever else you have eaten will reflect on the scale. Once you begin to eat healthy again, you will come back down in weight. Having a free day works for me right now. I usually take my free day on Saturday. By Sunday I am back on track. You can also do one free meal a week. This something a lot of people do. It helps them to indulge in just a little unhealthy food and not get carried away with eating a lot of junk food. When you are starting your healthy lifestyle journey, this may be the option you want to pick. Or, you can have a free meal every other week.

What is the benefit of having a free meal or free day per week? Personally, it helps me get through the cravings I may have during the week. It is my motivation to stick to the plan and eat healthy until that day comes. When I get a craving (they say a craving lasts around 30 minutes), I tell myself, "I can have that on Saturday." I wouldn't be honest if I didn't tell you that, sometimes I have given into these cravings. No one is perfect and this will happen sometimes. When it does, I don't beat myself up about it. I say, "Okay, I wasn't supposed to eat that." I get up, dust myself off, and when it is time to eat that next meal I get back on track. Please don't beat yourself up if you get off track. It isn't going to help. Just admit your mistake and move on and get back on track.

"Lucky thing opportunity is never on vacation, never in short supply." *Kenroy G.*

One way to avoid giving into cravings or temptation is to prep your food for the week, or at least for a couple of days, and to take it with you when you leave the house. On Sunday, I cook my meals for the next five days. It is an all day process, but I cook all of my lunch and dinner for those five days. I like to eat my breakfast hot, so I will cook breakfast fresh every day. The key to prepping your meals is to make sure you have enough variety of foods to eat during the week. If you don't have a variety of meals, you will become bored with eating the same food every day. If you don't want to eat what you have cooked for the week, you may end up turning to unhealthy foods.

You may be worried that this is very time consuming. But when you cook all your meals ahead of time on one day, that frees up the time in the next few days that you would put into thinking about what to cook, as well as the time spent defrosting, preparing, and then cooking the food. Once you cook your meals for the week, put them in Tupperware dishes, for each day. For each day of the week in my refrigerator, I have containers for my morning snack, lunch, afternoon snack and dinner. In the morning before leaving to go to work, I grab my Tupperware containers and place them in my lunch bag. If I am home I pull my meal out of the refrigerator, heat it up and then eat it.

Have you ever been hungry while cooking, then you start to snack while preparing your meal? If your food is prepped for you, when you get hungry, you can take it out of the refrigerator and eat it. This will stop you from eating extra calories.

———◈———

""No Matter what you do in Life the condition of your health will determine how well you do it." Leonard V.

———◈———

If you have a family like mine, where everyone isn't eating as healthy as you are, prepping your food and eating it before you start cooking helps you to not munch on their food as you make it. You should be already full from eating the food you prepped for yourself. I also can't stress enough the importance of staying hydrated and drinking liquids throughout the day. Sometimes, that "hunger" you feel may not be hunger at all. It could be that you are thirsty. If 30 minutes to 1 hour after you have eaten, you are hungry again, drink some water or tea to make sure you aren't thirsty. If, after drinking the water or tea, you are still hungry, eat a piece of fruit or a (small!) handful of nuts.

Before talking about the different types of foods you should eat, I want to tell you one tip again: Whenever you walk out of the house, take food with you! This is very important to fight cravings and temptations.

Before I started my healthy lifestyle journey, I would stop at McDonald's almost every day, sometimes even twice a day. I would eat the same thing every time: a filet of fish sandwich meal, no salt on my fries with an ice tea (½ sweetened and ½ unsweetened). One of the hardest habits for me to break was stopping at McDonald's when I was out if I got hungry. In the beginning I didn't take my food with me. This was a HUGE mistake. I had to fight the temptation of wanting to stop all the way home, which wasn't easy to do.

"It's your body OWWN it." Nicole N.

I learned I needed to start taking food with me when I left my house. Now, if I am out and get hungry, I have a piece of fruit or nuts, or celery and carrots, to eat instead of McDonalds. When leaving your house, you never know when you will be back home, even if you're only planning to go out for a specific time. Have you ever ended up being out all day unexpectedly and been so hungry that you stopped to pick up something unhealthy? Taking food with you will help to eliminate this issue.

What I Eat

Growing up, I ate three meals a day. So as an adult I also ate three meals a day. Once I started to exercise, I began to eat more food throughout the day, at meals and between. Not "bad" food, but not very healthy food either. When I decided to start living a healthy lifestyle, I began eating 5-6 meals a day. Eating five (to six) times a day can be an effective strategy for maintaining a healthy body weight, according to a 2011 study published in the *Journal of the American Dietetic Association*. It is believed that eating small meals (5-6) throughout the day can lower cholesterol, promote weight loss, improve energy levels, boost metabolism, and preserve lean muscle mass.

"Your passion is your driving force behind your success."
Zhivi W

As I've said, I eat 5 meals a day. I eat breakfast, lunch, dinner and two snacks. If I am up later than usual and I get hungry, I will eat a third snack. Usually my breakfast consists of oatmeal, egg whites and 1 whole egg, and turkey bacon (uncured). After eating breakfast I am full, not stuffed. In two to three hours I am ready to eat my first snack. I cycle through different snacks; for example, an apple with almond butter or a small amount of chicken breast and brown rice, or even a small salad. These snacks are a smaller amount than a meal would be. In two to three hours I am ready for lunch. Lunch is always a carb (brown rice), steamed or raw vegetables and a protein (usually chicken breast). Two to three hours later it is time for another snack and then dinner is another two to three hours after. My dinner usually consists of steamed or raw vegetables and protein. I don't eat carbs for dinner. If I get hungry after dinner, I eat a green apple before bed.

People have asked me, "Do you count calories?" The answer is no. I've counted calories in the past using a calorie counting online app, but for me it was too time consuming. (To be honest, I hated it.) Once I learned how to eat healthfully, and that I could eat as many vegetables as I wanted (they have a low calorie count), I was all too happy not to count calories any longer. If you eat a lot of vegetables and do not eat any carbs for dinner, there is no need to count calories at all to lose weight.

"The attitude of one can affect so many the faith of one can inspire the world". Phillip B.

As stated elsewhere, I also suggest that people have either a free day or a free meal. I personally have a free day where I will eat whatever I want. I would not suggest this if you are just starting your journey, or if you have a lot of weight to lose. To begin, I would suggest eating healthy for two weeks, then pick a day for a "free" meal. (I usually like to eat my free meal for lunch or dinner.) For a lot of people, it is hard to get back on track when having a free day. Know that you will gain weight if you take a free day and eat whatever you want. You can gain up to 3 pounds from one day. How? Processed foods, a lot of sugar or salt, all these things your body has gotten out of its system during healthy eating, will cause bloating and water retention. Not drinking a lot of water on your free day will also increase the amount of water weight you gain.

However, a free meal or a free day gives you the opportunity to eat whatever you have been craving during the week, or weeks. I find these days help me to stay on track. If I have a craving, I tell myself, "You can wait until Saturday to eat that." By the time my free meal or free day comes, I usually no longer want what I was craving but I am really in the mood for something else. There are even times where I will eat healthy on a free day because I don't want any unhealthy food!

A lot of people say that we eat with our eyes—as long as you see the food, you will eat the food. This is one reason why eating healthfully at a restaurant can be so hard. One strategy I use when I eat out, is to ask the waiter to bring me a to-go box along with my food. I will put half of the food in the to-go box to take home and only eat what I "see" on the plate. I also drink warm lemon water. Warm lemon water aids the digestive system and makes the process of eliminating the waste products from the body easier. It also helps to prevent the problem of constipation and diarrhea. Drinking cold drinks during meals, or after eating, can cause the food to become solid again in the stomach and thus hard to digest. Normally when you eat food, such as butter or some cheeses, the temperature in our stomach is warm enough to keep them in a semi liquid state. When eating a meal, drink something warm, like coffee (black), tea, warm water, or warm lemon water. Drinking warm liquids will aid in the digestion of a meal by softening the food in your stomach.

"Time to rebuild or finally create the world you've always wanted. You are more powerful than you imagine. STOP DOUBTING & START DOING"
Phillip B.

WHAT I PERSONALLY DO

I don't drink a lot of different things. I drink water, green and peppermint tea, and also warm lemon water. From time to time I may have a soda (pop) or a sweet tea. When I do drink sweet tea, I ask them to cut it half and half, sweet and unsweet, or sometimes I tell them, "more unsweet than sweet."

Five out of seven days a week I drink warm lemon water when I first wake up. When I first started drinking lemon water, I could not drink just lemon water. I had to put something in it. I drank lemon water with cucumbers in it to start. I slowly began to put fewer and fewer cucumbers in my water until now all I drink is warm lemon water. This may be something you want to try if you don't like drinking lemon water. I also have never used a lot of lemons; I tend to use one lemon per gallon of water.

I am always working toward drinking more water. Drinking water is my downfall—I never drink enough. At my best, I was drinking a gallon a day. But then I would fall back into not drinking maybe one-third of what I was supposed to be drinking. That isn't good at all, but it goes to show that no matter where you are on your healthy living

———◆———

" Being STRONG is a choice you must make DAILY."
Phillip B

———◆———

Abs are Made in the Kitchen

The flat stomach or 6-pack abs you are looking for will be made by what you eat. First, you need to create a decent calorie deficit to lower body fat. Food intake versus calories burned is the ticket. Here are a few rules to remember in the process of creating the stomach or abs you want:

1. Commit 100% to clean eating. Cheat meals are okay.
2. Cut out processed foods. Cook your own meals.
3. Cut out white flour. Use whole grain flour, sprouted grain flout, gluten free flour or brown rice flower.
4. Cut out refined sugar or salts. Us agave nectar, honey, brown rice syrup, sea or Himalayan salts.
5. Eat healthy fats. They speed up your body's fat burning ability to help you burn fat faster.
6. Add sources of lean protein such as chicken, fish and Greek yogurt.
7. Drink more water. Water flushes out toxins, excess water and sodium.

80% of your healthy diet and 20% of your workout will allow for you to get the stomach you are looking for. Healthy eating will lower the amount of body fat you have, while working out will strengthen your stomach muscle.

———◆———

"Your passion is your driving force behind your success."
Zhivi W

———◆———

My Top 11 Tips

If you put in the time and effort, staying focused and committed, you can lose weight and look the way you want. It may not be easy when you start—nothing usually is when doing something new—but if you stay committed, thing will get easier. Here are 11 tips to keep you on track with living a healthy lifestyle:

1. **Learn how to motivate and encourage yourself.** Motivation and encouragement from others is always great, but what happens when they aren't available? You have to find a way to motivate and encourage yourself. Find motivational sayings, bible verses, pictures of yourself or others—anything that will keep you focused. Then, when you feel like you don't want to exercise or to eat well, you can remember your motivational words or look at your pictures to keep going.

2. **Stop saying you're on a "diet."** When you make a commitment to start living a healthy lifestyle, it is permanent. The word "diet" to me means you start at a certain weight, lose weight to reach a goal, but have no plan after that. With no plan, what usually happens is you go back to eating the way you did before the journey, and now all the hard work, sweat and tears that you put into the "diet" has been wasted. You slowly start to gain weight back and usually end up weighing more than when you started. To avoid this, make a lifestyle change not a temporary switch.

3. **Find a workout that works for you.** Do what you like. Not everyone likes to lift weights. If you don't, don't. If you enjoy running, run; if you enjoy going to classes, then you should do that.

4. **Have a great support team.** This is so important. There are going to be times on this journey when your mind will try to sabotage what your progress. You don't need others in your corner doing the same thing; this can cause you to quit. Find people who are going through, or who have been through, the same journey you are on.

5. **Have fun.** Yes, you can have fun on a healthy lifestyle journey!

6. **Take pictures of yourself.** From seeing how I was doing during my weight loss journey to now monitoring how I am maintaining my shape, I take progress pictures and measurements every four weeks. The best part about this habit is that at the end of the year, I have a year's worth of pictures to see how I have improved. You may not see the difference at first, but as you take them you will begin to see the gradual changes in your body. Share them with people you know, even if you're shy. Honest people will tell you the changes they see, when you might not see them yourself. Take a front, back and side picture.

7. **Lead by example.** People are going to be watching you, especially if you share with them that you are now going to start living a healthy lifestyle. The more you stay focused and they see how you improve, the more they will begin to ask you questions and to change what they are doing to follow you.

8. **Get your family involved.** Not everyone will want to eat as healthfully as you will, so start them out slowly. If you are used to fixing canned veggies, start cooking frozen veggies, then move to fresh. Everyone loves some kind of

fruit—start leaving out more fruit in the house for them to eat as a snack.

9. **Research.** If you have been diagnosed with a medical condition, research the best diet for you. Read books on the medical condition you have, and go online to research the condition and find support groups. Buy some magazines for different exercises. If you use Facebook, join positive, encouraging groups that discuss about healthy eating. There are a number of them out there. If you get in a group and don't like what you see, leave that group and find another one.

10. **Please get your recommended hours of sleep, or close to it, and learn to relax**. This is important. Sleep deprivation can cause weight gain on top of other issues. Stop running from place to place, trying to do and be that person for everyone. That isn't your job. You need to take the time out for yourself, to relax your mind, body and spirit. A lot of running around, getting no sleep, and eating unhealthy food has its consequences—your body can shut down on you or become ill. Do it long enough, and other medical conditions, even heart attacks (This happened to somebody I know) can occur. You are one person; stop trying to save the world. Let some things go. If you are running every day, all day long, learn to tell people NO and take at least one day for yourself. Even God knew He needed to rest, which is why everything was created in six days, not seven. None of us are God, so why try to do something not even He did?

11. **When you do go out to eat with friends, family or alone, chose healthy dishes and ask how they are cooked.** This helps a lot. A lot of restaurants are willing to accommodate the way you want your food to be cooked. I have asked how a dish is cooked, whether I get it with no seasoning, with steamed vegetables on the side with no seasoning, etc. You

don't always have to eat a salad when you go out to eat unless you want one. Sometimes a salad, depending on what is in it and the amount of salad dressing you use, can be just as unhealthy as a burger and fries.

Recipes

The information in this chapter is not intended to replace the information from your doctor or a certified nutritionist. Always work directly with your doctor or a nutritionist before changing your diet and lifestyle. Always ask your doctor before making any changes in what you eat. Before consuming large quantities of anything you're not familiar with (or, if you have any special medical condition or are taking any prescription medication), please do some research and/or talk to your doctor.

When cooking your food, prepare it by steaming, baking, grilling or eating it raw (not meat). Fill the majority of your plate with vegetables. Eat fruit for dessert.

Breakfast

Salmon and Eggs with Spinach

Ingredients:
- 2 eggs or 3 egg whites
- 2 slice raw salmon
- 1 large handful spinach

Directions:
1. Pre-boil the eggs the night before to save time or poach them in the morning.
2. Cook salmon and steam spinach.
3. Place eggs, salmon and spinach on a plate.

Cooking Salmon

1. Preheat the oven to 425°F
2. Pat the salmon dry
3. Rub the salmon with oil, salt, and pepper
4. Place the salmon in the roasting pan
5. Roast for 4 to 6 minutes per half-inch thickness of salmon
6. Salmon is done when easily flaked

Organic Turkey Sausage Omelet

Ingredients:
- 2 natural turkey sausages (Natural Savory Turkey Breakfast Sausage)
- 3 eggs or 4 egg whites
- 5 asparagus spears
- 1 large handful spinach
- 2 large tomatoes

Directions
1. Pre-grill the sausages the night before to save time.
2. Crack eggs into a bowl and beat them.
3. Sauté asparagus, spinach and tomatoes in a pan.
4. Remove asparagus, spinach and tomatoes from the pan and set to the side.
5. Place raw scrambled eggs in the pan and add the sautéed vegetables to the eggs; cook 2-3 minutes.
6. Flip the omelet and let cook 2-3 minutes; place on plate.
7. Eat turkey sausage on the side.

RECIPES

Blueberry Almond Flour Pancakes

Ingredients:
- 1 cup almond flour
- 2 eggs
- 1/4 cup almond milk, or water
- Pinch salt
- Blueberries

Directions
1. Mix ingredients together.
2. Heat a pan on the stove with a little oil.
3. Sprinkle a few flecks of water into the pan. When water sizzles, add batter to the pan.
4. Cook for 2 minutes on each side or until you see bubbles form and pop around the edges of the batter.
5. Flip the pancake and cook for 2 minutes.
6. Remove and top with fruit or syrup.

Apple Oatmeal Pancakes

Ingredients:
- 6 egg whites
- 1/4 cup oatmeal (dry)
- 1 tablespoon unsweetened apple sauce
- Pinch of cinnamon powder
- Pinch of stevia
- 1 cup (4.4 oz.) apple, chopped finely
- 1/4 teaspoon baking soda
- Cooking spray

Directions
1. Mix ingredients together.
2. Heat a pan on the stove with a little oil.
3. Sprinkle a few flecks of water into the pan. When water sizzles, add batter to the pan.

4. Cook for 2 minutes or until you see bubbles form and pop around the edges of the batter.
5. Place some of the diced apple on the pancake.
6. Flip the pancake and cook for 2 minutes.
7. Remove and top with fruit or syrup.

Huevos Mexicanos

Ingredients:
- 6 egg whites
- 1 teaspoon olive oil
- 1/3 cup onion, chopped
- 1/2 tomato, diced
- 1/4 cup avocado sliced
- 1/4 cup fresh cilantro, chopped
- Pinch of chili powder

Directions
1. Beat the egg whites with chili powder. Set aside.
2. In a large skillet, heat oil over medium-high heat.
3. Add the chopped onion. Stir-fry until the onion is translucent.
4. Stir in seasoned eggs.
5. Scramble until eggs are almost fully cooked.
6. Add tomato, avocado and cilantro; stir in gently until everything is well mixed together.

Blueberry Bran Protein Muffins

Ingredients:
- 1 cup oat bran
- 1/2 cup flax meal
- 4 scoops protein powder, flavor of your choice (vanilla is the best to use)
- 2/3 cup frozen blueberries
- 1 teaspoon stevia
- 1 teaspoon cinnamon
- 1/4 teaspoon salt
- 1 teaspoon baking powder

- 3 egg whites
- 1 teaspoon maple extract
- 2/3 cup water

Directions:
1. In a big bowl, mix all the ingredients (except for the blueberries).
2. Stir until the mix gets thick.
3. Add the blueberries and stir (with a spoon or a spatula).
4. Scoop into a muffin pan coated with cooking spray.
5. Bake at 350°F for 25 minutes.

Club Omelet

Ingredients:
- 1 slice turkey bacon, cooked
- 2oz turkey or chicken breast
- 1/2 small tomato, diced
- 1 scallion, sliced
- 4 egg whites
- 1 egg
- 1oz low fat cheddar
- Pinch of sea salt
- Pinch of black pepper

1. Beat the eggs with the water and the soy sauce. Set aside.
2. In a large skillet, heat oil over medium-high heat.
3. Add the ginger, then the meat and remaining ingredients.
4. Stir-fry until the onion is translucent and the cabbage and bean sprouts are tender-crisp.
5. Stir in seasoned eggs.
6. Scramble until eggs are cooked.

Turkey Breakfast Sausage Patties

Ingredients:
- 1 lb ground turkey
- 1 teaspoon sea salt
- 2 teaspoons sage
- 1 teaspoon fennel seed
- 1 teaspoon thyme
- 1 teaspoon black pepper
- 1/2 teaspoon white pepper
- 1/2 teaspoon cayenne
- 1/4 teaspoon garlic powder
- 1/8 teaspoon ground cloves
- 1/8 teaspoon nutmeg
- 1/8 teaspoon allspice

Directions
1. Combine all ingredients (use less pepper if you don't want a spicy taste) and blend well.
2. Refrigerate overnight to let the meat absorb the flavor of the spices.
3. Form into patties and cook as needed, freezing leftovers.
4. Don't overcook or they will dry out—remove from the heat as soon as they're no longer pink inside, but still juicy.
5. If you prefer a moister texture, you can add a splash of olive oil or an egg to the mixture just prior to cooking,

Almond-Oat Granola Bars

Ingredients:
- 1 1/2 cups almonds or slivered regular almonds (no skin)
- 1/4 cup 100% pure maple syrup
- 1/4 cup packed light-brown sugar
- 2 1/2 teaspoons vanilla
- 1/4 teaspoon kosher salt
- 1/4 cup plus 1 tablespoon canola oil
- 2 cups old-fashioned oats

Directions
1. Preheat oven to 300 degrees. Line a rimmed baking sheet with a silicone baking mat or parchment paper.
2. In mini-prep food processor, pulse the almonds 15 times. If not using a food processor, roughly chop the almonds.
3. In a large bowl, whisk together the syrup, sugar, vanilla, salt and oil. Add the oats and nuts and stir it all together well, using a rubber spatula.
4. Turn the batter out onto the cookie sheet. Using a stiff metal spatula, gently press it into an even layer in the shape of a 9-by-13 rectangle. It should be even on the top and all sides.
5. Bake uncovered for 15 minutes. Cover with foil and bake another 15 minutes. Check the color. If not yet light golden brown and beginning to harden, take the foil off and bake another five minutes uncovered. Let cool for one hour. When cool, gently break into pieces and store in airtight container or plastic zip-top bag.

Note: The color should be light golden. If edges start turning darker brown, immediately remove from oven.

Variations:
*   Don't stop at granola bars: use these ideas for even healthier, convenient snacks!
*   **Hit-the-Trail Mix:** Crumble 1 cup granola into small pieces. Add 1 cup chopped nuts of choice, ¼ cup mini chocolate chips and ¼ cup dried raisins or cranberries, if desired.
*   **Plant Protein Bar:** Spread 1 tablespoon natural peanut butter or almond butter atop granola square and enjoy!

Beef

Easy Meatballs

Ingredients:

- 1 pound of extra lean (5% fat) ground beef (or any ground lean red meat)
- ½ cup of minced onion
- 2 egg whites
- 1 egg
- 1/4 cup oat bran
- 2 tablespoons low fat parmesan
- 1 teaspoon oregano
- 1/2 teaspoon garlic powder
- 1 teaspoon of dried parsley
- 2 tablespoons of skim milk
- Salt and pepper

Directions
1. In a large bowl, mix all the ingredients together.
2. Shape into balls, 20 meatballs total.
3. Bake for 25 minutes at 375°F.

Stuffed Peppers

Ingredients:

- 8oz extra lean (5% fat) ground beef (or any ground lean red meat)
- 1 cup cooked brown rice
- 1 onion, finely chopped
- 1/4 cup grated low fat parmesan cheese
- 3 garlic cloves, minced
- 1/2 teaspoon dried thyme
- 1/2 teaspoon dried basil
- 4 green, red, or yellow bell peppers, tops cut off and seeded
- 1/2 cup tomato puree or tomato sauce

Directions
1. Preheat oven to 350°F.
2. Mix together beef, rice, onion, parmesan, tomato sauce, garlic, thyme, and basil in large bowl then spoon evenly into bell peppers.
3. Stand peppers in shallow baking dish or casserole.
4. Pour tomato puree over peppers and add enough water to baking dish to come partway up sides of peppers.
5. Cover baking dish with foil and bake, basting peppers and rice are tender and filling is cooked through, about 20 minutes longer.
6. Let stand 5 minutes before serving.

Sweet Pepper Beef Stir-Fry

Ingredients:
- 8oz lean red meat
- 1 tablespoon coconut oil
- 1 tablespoon lemon juice
- 1 cup broccoli florets
- 1 teaspoon garlic
- 1/2 cup onion, chopped
- 1 teaspoon dried parsley
- 1 teaspoon dried oregano
- 1/4 cup low-sodium beef broth
- 1 carrot; cut in thin wedges
- 1 green bell pepper; cut in wedges
- 1 red bell pepper; cut in wedges
- 1 orange bell pepper; cut in wedges

Directions
1. Thinly slice the meat across the grain.
2. Put the oil in a wok or skillet over high heat. When it's hot, add the beef and stir-fry for about 3-4 minutes.
3. Add red, green and orange pepper, garlic, broccoli, carrot, lemon juice and onion, stir-fry for 1 minute.

4. Add parsley and oregano, stir fry for another minute.
5. Add broth.
6. Stir until sauce thickens.

Chicken and Turkey

Chicken Almond Stir-Fry

Ingredients:
- 2 boneless, skinless chicken breasts (4oz each), cooked and cut into cubes
- 1 tablespoon soy sauce
- 1/4 cup low sodium chicken broth
- 1 clove garlic, crushed
- 1 teaspoon fresh ginger, grated
- 2 teaspoons coconut oil
- 1/4 cup slivered almonds
- 1 cup broccoli florets
- 1 cup snow peas; cut in half
- 1 cup mushrooms, sliced
- 2 scallions; cut into pieces about 1 inch (2.5 cm) long

Directions
1. Stir together the soy sauce, broth, garlic, and ginger.
2. Heat 1 teaspoon of coconut oil in a wok or large skillet over high heat
3. Add the almonds and stir-fry them until they're light golden.
4. Remove and set aside.
5. Heat another teaspoon of coconut oil in the pan and add the broccoli, snow peas, mushrooms, and scallions to the pan.
6. Stir-fry for about 5 minutes or until just barely tender-crisp.
7. Add the chicken and stir-fry for about 1 minute and toss everything together well.
8. Cover and simmer for 3 to 4 minutes. Top with the almonds and serve.

Chicken Burritos

Ingredients:
- 2 cooked chicken breasts (4oz each)
- 1 clove garlic, crushed
- 1/2 teaspoon chili powder
- 1 teaspoon olive oil
- 1 teaspoon lime juice
- 1 jalapeño, minced (optional)
- 2 small tortillas
- 1/2 cup shredded lettuce
- 1/4 cup fat free shredded cheddar cheese
- 2 tablespoons salsa
- Chopped fresh cilantro (optional)

Directions
1. In a bowl, mix the garlic, chili powder, oil, lime juice, salt, and jalapeño together.
2. Add chicken and stir.
3. Fill each tortilla with ½ mixture and top with lettuce, cheese, 1 tablespoon sour cream, 1 tablespoon salsa, and a sprinkling of cilantro.
4. Wrap and eat.

Chicken and Cucumber Toss

Ingredients:
- Baked and shredded chicken
- Cucumber; chopped
- Tomato; chopped
- Italian Dressing (look under the dressing section)
- Fresh, Italian parsley for garnish

Directions:
1. Toss as much of each ingredient together as you like in a mixing bowl and serve.

Chicken Vindaloo

Ingredients:
- 4 boneless, skinless, chicken breasts (4 oz. each)
- 1/4 cup onion, chopped
- 1 clove garlic, crushed
- 1 tablespoon grated ginger
- 1/2 teaspoon cumin
- 1/2 teaspoon coriander
- 1 teaspoon turmeric
- 2 tablespoons lime juice
- 2 tablespoons apple cider vinegar
- 1/2 cup low sodium chicken broth (or make your own)
- Pinch of cinnamon, salt, pepper

Directions
1. Put the chicken, onion, and garlic in a slow cooker.
2. In a bowl, stir together the remaining ingredients.
3. Pour the mixture over the chicken.
4. Cover the slow cooker, set it to low, and let it cook for 6 to 7 hours.

Turkey Spinach Zucchini Ravioli

Ingredients:
- 1.5 lbs. ground turkey
- 2 cups chopped fresh spinach
- 1/2 large onion
- 2 cloves of garlic
- 2 tsp. of Grill Mates- Montreal Chicken Seasoning (or you could use just salt & pepper)
- Zucchini
- Tomato Marinara Sauce of your choice

Directions
1. Slice zucchini with peeler; set strips aside.
2. In a medium wok combine: ground turkey, chopped fresh

spinach, 1/2 large onion, 2 cloves of garlic, and seasoning; sauté until turkey is cooked all the way through

3. Assemble the "ravioli" using 4 zucchini strips and 2 tbsp. of turkey mixture.
4. Wrap the zucchini around the turkey mixture and put face down in baking dish.
5. Top with marinara sauce and bake at 350F for approx. 30 minutes

Seafood

Curried Shrimp Kabobs

Ingredients:
- 24 jumbo cooked frozen shrimp
- 1 tsp garlic (finely minced)
- 1/4 tsp curry powder
- 1/2 tsp turmeric
- 1/4 tsp cumin
- Sea salt and pepper, to taste
- 16–20 cherry tomatoes
- 2 large yellow onions, cut into large chunks
- 8 large wooden skewers (soaked in water for 10 minutes)

Directions
1. Preheat tabletop grill or outdoor grill.
2. In a large bowl or large Ziploc bag, mix curry powder, turmeric, cumin, salt, pepper and garlic.
3. Add shrimp and onions to spice mixture. Coat shrimp and onions thoroughly, being careful not to break up the onion chunks.
4. Thread 3 shrimp onto each skewer, alternating with tomatoes and onions.
5. Spray grill with non-stick cooking spray and cook until

brown and onions are tender, about 8 minutes (flip halfway through if using outdoor grill).

Optional: Serve over brown rice.

Fish Sticks

Ingredients:
- 2 tilapia fillets (4oz each)
- 1 egg
- 1 teaspoon coconut oil
- 1 tablespoon low fat parmesan
- 1/3 cup oatmeal (ground)
- 1 teaspoon onion powder
- 1/2 teaspoon dried parsley
- Salt and pepper

Directions
1. Preheat oven to 375°F. Prepare baking sheet by coating with coconut oil.
2. Cut each tilapia filet into 3 equal sticks (you should have 6 sticks total).
3. Set aside.
4. Grind oatmeal in a food processor (or blender).
5. Combine the parmesan, onion powder, dried parsley, and a pinch of salt and pepper in a large container with a tightly fitting lid. Shake well. This is your coating mixture.
6. Add egg in a medium bowl.
7. Dip each stick in the egg-whites. Then dip each stick in the coating mixture. Make sure each piece is well coated.
8. Place on the baking sheet. When all of your fish has been coated and your baking sheet is full, place in the oven and bake for 10 minutes or until golden.
9. Then flip the sticks and bake for an additional 5-6 minutes.

Orange Citrus Shrimp over Mixed Greens

Ingredients
- 10 cups (2 bags) spring mix
- 4 cups radicchio
- 4 cups arugula
- 2 cups Belgian endive
- 1/4 cup black olives, pitted (optional)
- 1 lb. shrimp
- 1 seedless orange, peeled and sliced
- Orange Citrus Dressing (get recipe from the dressings section)

Directions:
1. Place spring mix, radicchio, arugula, Belgian endive, and black olives in a large mixing bowl and set aside.
2. Grill or broil shrimp until they appear white.
3. Whisk together ingredients for Orange Citrus dressing in a small bowl and add a salad, tossing gently.
4. Place greens on serving dish and top with cooked shrimp; garnish with orange slice.

Salmon Hash

Ingredients:
- 8oz salmon; cooked
- 2 teaspoon olive oil
- 1/4 cup chopped onions
- 1/4 cup chopped green bell peppers
- 1/4 cup chopped red bell peppers
- 1 clove garlic; crushed
- 1 medium sweet potato, skinless, diced and cooked

Directions
1. Heat oil in skillet over medium-high heat.
2. Sauté onion, bell peppers, and garlic in oil.
3. Stir in potatoes and salmon.
4. Cook uncovered, stirring frequently, until hot.

Desserts

Banana Ice Cream

Ingredient:
- 4 bananas

Directions:
1. Peel your bananas.
2. Cut them into small pieces.
3. Freeze overnight in a plastic bag.
4. Let them thaw a little before making the ice cream.
5. Blend in the food processor, scraping down the bowl when they stick.
6. Place mixture in a freezable bowl
7. If you would like a more solid mixture, freeze for a couple of hours, then eat and enjoy.

Banana, Peach Almond Meal Ice Cream

Ingredient:
- 4 bunch bananas
- 2 peaches
- 1/4 cup almond meal (finely ground almonds)

Directions:
1. Peel your bananas.
2. Cut them into small pieces.
3. Freeze overnight in a plastic bag.
4. Let them thaw a little before making the ice cream.
5. Blend in the food processor, scraping down the bowl when they stick.

6. Place mixture in a freezable bowl
7. If you would like a more solid mixture, freeze for a couple of hours, then eat and enjoy.

Banana and Cacao Chip Ice Cream

Ingredient:
- 4 bunch bananas
- Cacao Chips

Directions:
1. Peel your bananas. Cut them into small pieces.
2. Freeze overnight in a plastic bag.
3. Let them thaw a little before making the ice cream.
4. Blend in the food processor, scraping down the bowl when they stick.
5. Place mixture in a freezable bowl.
6. Stir in cacao chips (be careful because these are strong).
7. If you would like a more solid mixture, freeze for a couple of hours, eat and enjoy.

Salad Dressings

Balsamic Vinaigrette

Ingredients:
- 1 tablespoon dried basil
- 1/4 cup balsamic vinegar
- 1/3 cup finely chopped shallots
- 1/3 cup water
- 1 tablespoon olive oil
- Pinch black pepper

Directions
1. Place of the all ingredients in a blender, blend until smooth

Creamy Dijon Herb

Ingredients:
- 4 tablespoons Greek yogurt
- 1/4 cup white wine vinegar
- 1/4 cup water
- 2 tablespoons minced fresh parsley
- 2 tablespoons Dijon mustard
- 1 tablespoon fresh lemon juice
- 1 garlic clove, minced
- 1 teaspoon dried thyme
- Pinch black pepper

Directions:
1. Place of the all ingredients in a blender and blend until smooth.

Italian Dressing

Ingredients:
- 1 cup apple cider vinegar
- 1 1/4 cup extra virgin olive oil
- 1 tbsp. garlic powder
- 1 tbsp. onion powder
- 1 tbsp. Italian herb
- 1 tsp. Dijon mustard, no sugar added
- 1 tsp. dried basil
- 1/2 tsp. ground black pepper
- 1/4 tsp. sea salt
- 1 tsp. honey (optional)

Directions
1. Combine all ingredients together in a medium mixing bowl and whisk well to combine.
2. Transfer the dressing to a storage container.
3. Keep in refrigerator for up to about 2 months.

Note: It is best to let this sit for 24 hours before using for the first time. This gives the herbs time to infuse into the oil. Shake well before every use.

Orange Citrus Dressing

Ingredients:
- 1 tbsp. shallots, minced
- 1/2 tsp orange zest, freshly grated
- 1/2 cup orange juice (fresh squeezed is better than store bought)
- 1/4 cup apple cider vinegar
- 1 tbsp. extra-virgin olive oil
- 1 tsp fresh oregano, chopped
- Pinch of Himalayan salt

Directions
1. Whisk together ingredients for Orange Citrus dressing in a small bowl.

Roasted Red Pepper Dressing

Ingredients:
- 1 1/2 tablespoons vegetable broth
- 1 tablespoon red wine vinegar
- 1 1/2 teaspoons olive oil
- 1/2 teaspoon salt
- 1/2 teaspoon Dijon mustard
- 1/4 teaspoon dried thyme
- 1/4 teaspoon black pepper
- 2 (7-ounce) bottles roasted red bell peppers, drained

Directions
1. Place all ingredients in a blender and process until smooth.
2. Refrigerate dressing in an airtight container for up to 1 week.

Shallot and Grapefruit Dressing

Ingredients:
- 1 teaspoon olive oil
- 1/2 cup chopped shallots
- 2 cups fresh grapefruit juice (about 3 grapefruits)
- 2 tablespoons chopped fresh cilantro
- 2 teaspoons sugar (honey or Stevia)
- 1/4 teaspoon freshly ground black pepper
- 2 tablespoons olive oil

Directions:
1. Heat 1 teaspoon oil in a large nonstick skillet over medium heat. Add shallots; cook 5 minutes or until golden brown. Stir in juice.
2. Bring to a boil over medium-high heat, and cook until reduced to 1 cup (about 6 minutes). Remove from heat; cool.
3. Place the grapefruit juice mixture, cilantro, sugar, and pepper in a blender; process until smooth. With blender on, slowly add 2 tablespoons oil. Process until smooth.

Sun-Dried Tomato Vinaigrette

Ingredients:
- 1/3 cup sun-dried tomatoes
- 1/4 cup red wine vinegar
- 1 tablespoon olive oil
- 1 garlic clove, minced

Directions:
1. Place of the all ingredients in a blender, blend until smooth.

Flavored Water

Citus

Ingredients:
- 1 orange
- 1 lime
- 1 lemon
- Ice
- Mint leaves
- Spoon

Directions:
1. Slice up one of each: orange, lime and lemon.
2. Use the spoon to squish them slightly, releasing some of the juices but not too much; you just want the flavor, not sour water.
3. Add in some mint leaves as you like.
4. Add in ice, fill it to the top of the jar and followed by water and stir.
5. Chill it in the fridge overnight and it'll be ready to drink the next day.

Raspberry Lime

Ingredients:
- 2 limes
- 2 cups raspberries
- Spoon

Directions
1. Slice two limes into half and squeeze the juices into the jar.
2. Add raspberries.
3. Use the spoon to slightly squish them again, add ice and water. Stir and refrigerate.

Blackberry Sage

Ingredients
- Sage
- 2 cups blackberries
- Spoon

Directions
1. Take a bunch of sage leaves and crush them by folding and pressing the spoon against them to release some of its flavor.
2. Add it into the jar with the blackberries.
3. Use the spoon to slightly squish them, add water & ice. Stir and refrigerate.

Watermelon Rosemary

Ingredients:
- Rosemary
- 2 cups cubed watermelon
- Ice
- Spoon

Directions
1. Slightly squish some rosemary at the bottom of the jar—these herbs release a strong flavor so not much pressing needed.
2. Add cubed watermelon and squish with the spoon gently.
3. Add water & ice, stir and refrigerate.

Homemade Pineapple Juice with a Cinnamon Twist

Ingredients:
- 1 whole pineapple
- 10-12 cups of water
- 1-2 cinnamon sticks
- 10-15 cloves
- 1/2-3/4 cup brown sugar, or whatever sweetener you like (optional)

Directions

1. Cut off the pineapple skin and cut the pineapple in half.
2. Cut out the core.
3. Combine the skin and core into a large pot with water.
4. Bring to a boil and simmer partly covered for about an hour, stirring occasionally.
5. Let cool down, then strain.
6. Refrigerate to allow the spices and pineapple flavor to concentrate.
7. It's quick and easy and a new way to enjoy pineapple juice.

Seasoning

Spice rub for any meat

Ingredients:

- 3 tablespoons dried minced onion flakes
- 2 tablespoons garlic powder
- 2 tablespoons dried orange peel
- 1 tablespoon ground black pepper
- 2 teaspoons dried parsley
- 1 teaspoon dried basil
- 1 teaspoon coriander
- 1 teaspoon cumin
- 1 teaspoon dried marjoram
- 1 teaspoon dried mustard
- 1 teaspoon dried oregano
- 1 teaspoon dried thyme
- 1 teaspoon cayenne pepper
- 1/2 teaspoon celery seed
- 1/2 teaspoon ground dried rosemary

BBQ

Ingredients:

- 1 tablespoon garlic powder
- 1 tablespoon celery seed
- 1 tablespoon onion powder
- 2 tablespoons paprika
- 1 tablespoon chili powder
- 2 teaspoons pepper

Cajun

Ingredients:

- 1 tablespoon thyme
- 2 teaspoons garlic powder
- 2 teaspoons dried onion flakes
- 1 teaspoon cumin
- 1 tablespoon paprika
- 1 teaspoon marjoram
- 1 teaspoon fennel
- 1/2 teaspoon of cayenne
- 1 teaspoon lemon pepper
- 1 teaspoon sage
- 1 teaspoon dried mustard
- 1/2 teaspoon dried thyme
- 1/2 teaspoon cayenne
- 1/4 teaspoon ground cloves

Chicken and fish

Ingredients:

- 2 tablespoons sesame seeds
- 1 teaspoon garlic powder
- 1 teaspoon dried onion flakes
- 1 teaspoon black pepper
- 1 teaspoon celery seed
- 1 teaspoon lemon zest (dried)
- 1 teaspoon dry mustard
- 1 teaspoon red pepper flakes

Curry

Ingredients:

- 1 tablespoon curry powder
- 1 teaspoon onion powder
- 1 teaspoon garlic powder

Fish and Seafood

Ingredients:
- 1 tablespoon celery seed
- 1 tablespoon black pepper
- 1/2 teaspoon ginger
- 5 ground bay leaves
- 1/2 teaspoon dry mustard
- 1 teaspoon paprika
- 1/4 teaspoon cinnamon

Herb

Ingredients:
- 3 tablespoons dried basil
- 3 tablespoons dried parsley
- 3 tablespoons dried oregano
- 3 tablespoons dried rosemary

Taco

Ingredients:
- 2 tablespoons chili powder
- 1/2 teaspoon garlic powder
- 1 teaspoon dried onion
- 1/2 teaspoon crushed red pepper flakes
- 1/2 teaspoon dried oregano
- 1 teaspoon paprika
- 1 1/2 teaspoons ground cumin
- 1 1/2 teaspoons cumin seed
- 1 teaspoon sea salt
- 2 teaspoon black pepper

Directions
1. Mix all ingredients.
2. Store in an airtight container.
3. This recipe will season approximately three pounds of meat, depending on how much you use.

Vegetable

Ingredients:
- 4 tablespoons dried parsley
- 2 tablespoons dried chives
- 1 teaspoon dried basil
- 1 teaspoon dried marjoram
- 1 teaspoon dried oregano
- 1 teaspoon dried thyme
- ½ teaspoon celery seed

Smoothies

Banana, Nectarine, Pineapple Green Smoothie

Ingredients
- 1 banana, peeled
- 1 nectarine
- 1/2 cup pineapples chopped
- Handful raw spinach

Directions
1. Add all the ingredients to the blender and blend on high for 30 seconds or until the smoothie is creamy.
2. If you would like more liquid add more pineapples. Place in the freezer to cool.

Beet Smoothie

Ingredients:
- 1 beet, chopped
- 2 oranges, peeled and deseeded
- 1 cup pineapples, cubed
- 1 banana, peeled
- 1 cup dandelion greens, chopped
- 4 ounces of filtered water

Directions
1. Add all the ingredients except for the greens to your blender and hit the "pulse" button a few times until you have a rough blend.
2. Add the greens and blend on high for 30 seconds or until the smoothie is creamy.

Blueberry "Milkshake"

Ingredients
- 2 frozen banana, peeled
- 4 ounces of vanilla hemp or almond milk
- 1 cup frozen blueberries

Directions:
1. Add all the ingredients and blend on high for 30 seconds or until the smoothie is creamy.

Carrot-Apricot Smoothie

Ingredients:
- 6 apricots, peeled and pitted
- 2 medium carrots or 1 cup grated/shredded
- 1 mango, peeled and pitted
- 4 to 6 ounces of filtered water

Directions
1. Add all the ingredients to your blender and blend on high for 30 seconds or until the smoothie is creamy.

Cucumber-Kiwi Green Smoothie

Ingredients:
- 1 large cucumber, chopped
- 3 kiwifruits, peeled
- 1 pear, cored
- 1/2 bunch of Swiss chard, chopped
- 1/2 head of romaine lettuce, chopped
- 4 ounces of filtered water

Directions
1. Add all the ingredients except for the greens to your blender and hit the "pulse" button a few times until you have a rough blend.
2. Add the greens and blend on high for 30 seconds or until the smoothie is creamy.

Green Apple, Peach, Banana Green Smoothie

Ingredients:
- 1 banana
- 1 peach
- 1/2 green apple
- Handful spinach
- Pineapple
- Chia seeds

Directions
1. Add all the ingredients to the blender and blend on high for 30 seconds or until the smoothie is creamy. If you would like more liquid add more pineapples.
2. Put a teaspoon of chia seeds in the smoothie after all ingredients have been blended together.
3. Place in the freezer to cool.

Orange-Ginger Smoothie

Ingredients:
- 2 oranges, peeled and deseeded
- 1 inch ginger, grated
- 1 pear, cored
- 1/2 head romaine lettuce, chopped
- 1/2 cup (4 ounces) rice milk

Directions
1. Add all the ingredients except for the greens to your blender and hit the "pulse" button a few times until you have a rough blend.
2. Add the greens and blend on high for 30 seconds or until the smoothie is creamy.

Raspberry and Goji Berry Smoothie

Ingredients:
- 1 cup raspberries
- 1 large mango, peeled and pitted
- 2 cups fresh baby spinach, chopped (or other leafy green)
- 4 ounces of almond milk
- 2 tablespoons goji berries, soaked for 20 minutes

Directions
1. Add all the ingredients except for the greens to your blender and hit the "pulse" button a few times until you have a rough blend.
2. Add the greens and blend on high for 30 seconds or until the smoothie is creamy.

Strawberry-Mango with a Hint of Pineapple Smoothie

Ingredients:

- 2 1/2 cups whole strawberries
- 1 cup pineapple, cubed
- 1 large ripe mango, peeled and pitted
- 1/2 head romaine lettuce, chopped
- 4 to 6 ounces of filtered water

Directions

1. Add all the ingredients except for the greens to your blender and hit the "pulse" button a few times until you have a rough blend.
2. Add the greens and blend on high for 30 seconds or until the smoothie is creamy.

Strawberry-Pineapple Smoothie

Ingredients:

- 1 cup pineapple, cubed
- 1 cup strawberries (fresh or frozen)
- 1 small peach, pitted
- 1 teaspoon flax seed
- 2 cups fresh spinach, chopped
- 4 to 6 ounces of almond milk

Directions

1. Add all the ingredients except for the spinach to your blender and hit the "pulse" button a few times until you have a rough blend.
2. Add the spinach and blend on high for 30 seconds or until the smoothie is creamy.

NOTE: If you don't have a high-speed blender, you'll want to grind the flax seeds in a coffee grinder before adding them to your smoothie.

Vegetables

Black Bean and Sweet Potato Chili

Ingredients:
- 1 small onion, diced
- 2 small sweet potatoes, peeled and chopped
- 2 medium carrots, sliced
- 1 red bell pepper, chopped
- 2 tablespoon olive oil
- 30oz can black beans (or make your own)
- 15oz can diced tomatoes (or chop your own)
- 1/2 cup low sodium vegetable broth (or make your own)
- 1 tablespoon chili powder
- 1 teaspoon cumin
- 1/2 teaspoon cayenne (or to taste)
- 1/2 teaspoon garlic powder
- Salt and pepper (Himalayan pink salt)

Directions
1. Sautee onions and garlic in olive oil for a minute or two, then add sweet potatoes, carrots and bell pepper until onions are soft, about 5-6 minutes.
2. Reduce heat to medium low, and add remaining ingredients, stirring to combine well.
3. Simmer, partially covered and stirring occasionally, for 20-25 minutes, until flavors have mingled and vegetables are cooked.

Cuban Black Beans

Ingredients:
- 1.5 cups black beans, rinsed and drained (or make your own)
- 1/2 cup red onion, chopped
- 1/2 cup green bell pepper, chopped
- 1 clove garlic, minced
- 1 bay leaf, finely chopped
- 1/2 teaspoon paprika
- 1/2 teaspoon cumin
- 2 tablespoons low sodium chicken broth (or make your own)
- 2 tablespoons red wine vinegar
- Salt and pepper

Directions
1. In a bowl, combine all the ingredients, mix well.

Curried Eggplant

Ingredients:
- 1 eggplant, sliced
- 1 teaspoon turmeric
- 1/2 teaspoon ginger
- (powder)
- Pinch of cayenne pepper
- Pinch of cinnamon

Directions
1. Coat a baking sheet with a light coat of cooking spray.
2. Lay eggplant slices on baking sheet.
3. In a bowl, mix all the spices together and sprinkle over eggplant slices.
4. Roast at 400°F for about 8 minutes.

Guacamole

Ingredients:
- 2 medium ripe avocados, peeled, de-pitted and largely diced (reserve the pits).
- 2 tbsp-1/4 cup finely diced onion (adjust amount according to how strong onions flavor is)
- 1 tbsp. cilantro, chopped (optional)
- 1-2 tbsp. fresh lime juice
- 1 medium or two small segments of garlic, crushed
- 2/3 cup diced Roma or plum tomatoes
- Salt (pink Himalayan) and pepper to taste

Directions:

This recipe involves making guacamole in a Ziploc bag. If you prefer you can, of course, smash the avocados with a fork and mix it in a bowl by hand.

1. In a gallon size Ziploc Bag combine all ingredients.
2. Seal bag and using your hands mush together until things are blended to your preferred consistency.
3. Taste guacamole and add salt and pepper and more lime juice if needed.
4. Clip edge of bag and squeeze into serving bowl.
5. Place pit or pits into the prepared guacamole, this will keep it looking fresh longer.

Kale Chips

Ingredients:
- 2 handfuls kale leaves
- 1 teaspoon cayenne pepper
- Cooking spray
- Sea salt

Directions
1. Preheat oven to 350°F.
2. Arrange kale on a nonstick baking sheet.
3. Very lightly coat kale with cooking spray and a bit of sea salt.
4. Sprinkle cayenne pepper on top of the kale and bake for 10 minutes or until crispy.

Louisiana Style Red Bean

Ingredients:
- 2 cups red kidney beans, rinsed and drained
- 1/2 cup red onion, chopped
- 1 clove garlic, minced
- 1 bay leaf
- Pinch of cayenne pepper
- Salt

Directions
1. In a large pot, combine beans with onion, garlic, salt, bay leaf, and cayenne pepper and cover with water.
2. Bring to boil, reduce heat and simmer for about 10 minutes or until done.

Quinoa Burritos

Ingredients:
- 2 small whole grain tortillas
- 1 whole egg
- 1/2 cup quinoa, cooked
- 4 egg whites
- 1/4 avocado, cubed
- 1 cup lettuce, shredded
- 1/4 cup salsa
- 1/4 cup red onion, diced
- 1/2 cup black beans
- 1/4 cup fresh cilantro

Directions
1. Cook quinoa (according the directions on the container) and eggs separately. Then mix with black beans, cilantro and onion.
2. Spread half mixture equally on whole wheat tortillas.
3. Top with salsa, avocado and lettuce.
4. Wrap and enjoy!

Spiced Summer Vegetable Casserole

Ingredients:
- 1.5 lbs. (about two) zucchini, sliced on a diagonal into half-inch pieces
- 1 lb. (about two) sweet potatoes, unpeeled, sliced on a diagonal into half-inch pieces
- 3/4 lb. (about two) beets, unpeeled, sliced into half-inch pieces
- 1 onion, sliced into 1/4-inch rounds
- 2 Tbsp. + 2 tsp. extra-virgin olive oil
- 2 tsp. balsamic vinegar 3/4 tsp. sea salt
- 1/2 tsp. garam masala chili flakes, to taste

Directions
1. Preheat oven to 375 degrees F.
2. Grease a large casserole dish with 2 tsp. of the olive oil.
3. Begin layering the vegetables, alternating between the zucchini, sweet potatoes, beets, and onion, starting on the outside and working your way in until you have an accordion-type pattern.
4. Drizzle with remaining 2 tbsp. olive oil. Sprinkle salt, garam masala, and chili flakes evenly over the top. Cover with parchment, then aluminum foil. Bake for 30 minutes.

Remove parchment and foil. Bake, uncovered, for an additional 30 minutes.

5. Serve hot, room temperature, or cold.

Steamed Okra Mix

Ingredients:
- 2 cups okra, sliced
- 1 cup, green bell pepper, sliced
- 1 tomato, diced
- 1 cup onion; cut in wedges
- 1/4 cup low-sodium chicken broth (or make your own)

Directions
1. Over medium-high heat, put all the veggies in large skillet.
2. Pour chicken broth on top, stir once, and cover.
3. Steam for about 5 minutes.

Tex Mex Spaghetti Squash Boats

Ingredients:
- 2 medium spaghetti squash
- 1 small onion, finely chopped
- 4 garlic cloves, crushed
- 1 large bell pepper, diced
- 14 oz. red kidney or black bean beans, drained & rinsed (or make your own)
- 1/2 tsp chili powder
- 2 tbsp. diced canned chilies or jalapeños (or to taste)
- 1 cup tomato sauce (no salt added or make your own)
- 1/2 cup cilantro, finely chopped + more for garnish
- 1 + 1/2 cup Colby Jack/Tex Mex/Mozzarella cheese, shredded & divided (I prefer goat cheese)
- 1/4 tsp salt (Himalayan pink salt; use less than what the recipe calls for)
- 1/2 tsp freshly ground black pepper
- Olive Oil Cooking spray

Directions
1. Preheat oven to 375 degrees F. Cut squash in half and scoop out the seeds with a spoon. Lay skin side down on a rimmed baking sheet, lined with parchment paper, and sprinkle with salt and pepper. Bake for 45 mins or until soft to a touch with a fork.
2. In the meanwhile, preheat medium skillet on medium heat and spray with cooking spray. Add onion, garlic, bell pepper and sauté for 4 - 5 minutes or until golden brown, stirring occasionally. Add beans, chili powder, chilies/jalapeños, tomato sauce, cilantro and stir. Remove from heat and add 1/2 cup cheese. Stir again.
3. Remove baked spaghetti squash from the oven and let cool a few minutes. Fluff each squash "boat" with a fork releasing some of the strands, leaving the squash in a shell. Fill each "boat" with heaping 3/4 - 1 cup prepared bean/pepper etc. mixture and sprinkle with 1/4 cup cheese each. Bake for additional 10 minutes or until cheese is melted. Serve hot, garnished with extra cilantro.
4. Refrigerate covered for up to 3 days. Do not freeze.

Vegetarian Cakes

Ingredients:
- 1 can (15oz) black beans- drained, rinsed and mashed (or make your own)
- 2 cloves garlic, minced
- Salt and pepper
- 3 tablespoons onion, minced
- Pinch of chili powder
- 1 egg, beaten
- 1/4 cup oat bran

Directions
1. In a food processor, mix all the ingredients.
2. Form 4 patties with mixture.
3. In a skillet, cook patties over medium heat for about 4 minutes per side.

Zucchini Oven Fries

Ingredients:
- 1 big zucchini
- 1 tablespoon oregano
- 1 tablespoon cumin

Directions
1. Cut zucchini into 1/4 inch by 3 inch (about 1/2 cm by 7 cm) sticks, like French fries.
2. Preheat oven to 500°F.
3. Arrange zucchini on non-stick baking sheet.
4. Combine spices and sprinkle over the zucchini fries.
5. Place in very hot oven and cook 15 to 18 minutes.

Appendix

Food Additives You Should Not Eat

There are many common additives in food that you should avoid for good health. The information on the additives listed here could change based on new studies and findings, so please do your own research in addition to mine.

- **Acesulfame-potassium** (Acesulfame K, Ace K, Sunett, Sweet One, potassium 6-methyl-2, 2-dioxo-oxathiazin-4-olate). Artificial sweetener. Found in thousands of foods, typically in soft drinks and other beverages such as instant coffee and tea, gelatin and pudding desserts, syrups, baked goods, chewing gum. Limited animal studies from more than 2 decades ago indicate it may cause cancer.
- **Artificial coloring** (check the cereal you are eating or giving to your children to eat) (FD&C Blue No. 1, FD&C Blue No. 2, FD&C Green no. 3, FD&C Red No. 3, FD&C Red No. 40, FD&C Yellow No. 5, FD&C Yellow No. 6, Orange B, Citrus Red no. 2). Food coloring. Usually found in low-nutrition foods, may also be added to "natural" foods like salmon to provide a more consistent tone in case of natural color variability. Recent studies suggest that artificial colorings cause hyperactivity and/or attention deficit order (ADD) in children. Researchers at the National College of

Technology in Japan tested the toxicity of 39 currently used food additives in 8 mouse organs. They reported that dyes were very toxic, causing DNA damage in the stomach, colon, urinary bladder, and gut. There are 9 certified colorings approved for use in the US by the FDA. Seven are permitted for use in foods:

- o FD&C Blue No. 1 (Brilliant Blue FCF)
- o FD&C Blue No. 2 (Indigotine)
- o FD&C Green No. 3 (fast Green FCF)
- o FD&C Red No. 3 (Erythrosine)
- o FD&C Red No. 40 (Allura Red AC)
- o FD&C Yellow No. 5 (Tartrazine)
- o FD&C Yellow No. 6 (Sunset Yellow)

- **Aspartame** (NutraSweet, Tropicana Slim, Equal, Canderel, aspartyl-phenylalanie-1-methyl ester). Artificial sweetener. Found in thousands of consumer food products. Commonly found in soft drinks, in individual packets of condiment, or even in chewable vitamins. Not suitable for baked products because it breaks down in heat. Individuals with the inherited metabolic disorder that prevents them from metabolizing the amino acid phenylalanine (PKU) must avoid this sweetener. Methanol breaks down in the body to a number of toxic metabolites such as formaldehyde. Formaldehyde production may be linked to incidence of migraines in aspartame users. Animal studies have indicated that aspartame may cause negative health effects such as cancer. People have reported that it causes headaches, hallucinations, seizures, insomnia, and dizziness.

- **Butylated hydroxyanisole (BHA) Antioxidant.** Widely used in fat-containing products like meats (sausage, lunch meats) butter, lard, cereals, and baked goods. May have estrogen-like effects. Studies have demonstrated it causes cancer in rats, mice and hamsters.

- **Butylated hydroxytoluene (BHT) Antioxidant**. Acute, high doses (0.5-1.0 grams per kilogram - much higher than levels found in foods) have led to kidney and liver damage in male rats. Rats fed BHT at lower doses over a longer period of time developed enlarged livers and reduced liver enzyme activity. Has been linked to DNA damage in mouse gut.
- **Calcium bromate.** Dough conditioner. Used in baked products like bread, rolls, and buns. Contains bromate, which may cause allergic reactions in sensitive individuals.
- **Cochineal extract** (carmine). Artificial coloring. Red food coloring made from the eggs of the cochineal beetle. Used to give foods like confections, meat, and spices their red, pink or purple coloring. It is not always clearly labeled on food products, and is often listed as a "natural" additive. Potential for both to provoke (severe) allergic reactions. Avoid if allergic.
- **Cottonseed oil.** Oil made from seeds of the cotton plant. Downside for cotton crops is the high level of pesticides used on them and that they tend to be GMO (Genetically modified organism). Commonly added to snack foods like potato chips. High in inflammatory (omega-6) polyunsaturated fats.
- **Diacetyl**. Flavoring agent. A clear yellow-green liquid with a buttery odor that naturally occurs in products like alcoholic beverages, coffee, cheese, cocoa, and berries, but can also be made through fermentation of glucose. Used in a number products to carry flavors—particularly microwave popcorn, margarines, and oils—to impart the aroma of butter. When used as an artificial butter flavoring, it can be a respiratory hazard when heated to high temperatures and inhaled.
- **Gluten** (wheat gluten). Dough conditioner, nutrient, stabilizer, texturizer, thickener. Principle protein fraction from

wheat. Added to foods like breads, ice cream and condiments for a variety of functions, but mainly to give structure and texture. Individuals with celiac disease need to follow a gluten-free diet. Due to the high number of individuals with gluten intolerance, it may be best to avoid this additive.

- **Hydrolyzed vegetable protein** (HVP, hydrolyzed protein, hydrolyzed soy protein, hydrolyzed wheat protein, hydrolyzed whey protein, hydrolyzed casein, TVP, texturized vegetable protein). Flavor enhancer. Plant protein that has been broken down into amino acids. Incorporated into instant soups, meats, sauces, and beef stew because of its savory (umami) meat flavor. Contains 10-30% MSG. Classified on some food labels as a "natural flavoring." May cause reactions like headache. Gluten-sensitive individuals should avoid if the source is wheat. Individuals with soy, wheat, or mil allergies should avoid proteins from these sources. Also avoid if allergic to MSG.

- **Isoamyl acetate**. Flavoring agent (artificial). Fruity flavoring that occurs naturally in bananas and pears, but is usually synthesized and used in beverages, ice cream, candy, baked goods and flavored fruit sodas. Exposure to high amounts has resulted in headache, fatigue, increased pulse, and irritation of nose and throat.

- **Monosodium glutamate** (MSG). Flavor enhancer. Sodium complexed to the amino acid, glutamic acid. Used to enhance savory (umami) flavor in meats, sauces, spices, instant meals, and bouillon cubes. Some people are sensitive to MSG and may experience nerve-toxic effects like headaches, mood changes, numbness, nausea, weakness, and burning sensation in the upper body. Natural flavorings, gelatin, hydrolyzed yeast, yeast extract, soy extracts, and hydrolyzed vegetable protein all contain glutamate.

- **Neotame**. Artificial sweetener. Similar in structure to aspartame. <u>7,000-13,000 times sweeter than table sugar and about 40 times sweeter than aspartame. Found in soft drinks, bars powdered drink mixes, juices, chewing gum, bread, frozen desserts, baked goods and candies.</u>
- **Olestra**. Fat substitute. Formed by the mixture of fatty acids and sucrose. It has fat-like properties, thus is used as a fat substitute. <u>Products containing olestra had to carry an FDA-mandated warning about side effects (abdominal cramping and loose stools)</u> and had to contain additional levels of fat-soluble vitamins (A, D, E, K) due to their malabsorption. <u>May be used in savory/salty ready to eat snacks (potato chips, tortilla chips, cheese puffs, crackers), tortillas, and ready to heat unpopped popcorn kernels.</u> It has been suggested that its consumption may worsen symptoms of irritable bowel syndrome (IBS). The Center for Science in the Public Interest opposes the use of olestra and accepts consumer complaints at http://www.cspinet.org/olestraform/index.htm
- **Partially hydrogenated oil** (partially hydrogenated cottonseed oil, partially hydrogenated palm oil, partially hydrogenated soybean oil, partially hydrogenated vegetable oil). Fat. As a result of hydrogenation, harmful trans fats are formed. Trans fats occur in small amounts in nature, such as in meats and milk. "Trans" refers to the chemical structure of the fat. <u>Partially hydrogenated oil is found in a multitude of processed food items: dessert and breads mixes, pastries, cookies, donuts, cake, crackers, frozen meals, French fries, margarines, shortening, taco shells, and microwave popcorn.</u> Eating these fats can have serious adverse health outcomes—probably more than any other fat, including saturated fat. <u>They increase the risk for heart disease by increasing bad (LDL) cholesterol and decreasing good (HDL) cholesterol.</u>

- **Potassium bromate**. Dough conditioner. White crystals or powder used to improve the function of flour in products like bread, rolls, and buns. Potassium bromate has been shown to cause cancer in animals and be toxic in human cells. Banned in Europe, Canada, China, Sri Lanka, Nigeria, Brazil and Peru. Not banned in the US. If used in a product in California, label must carry a cancer warning. Present in a product if "bromated flour" is listed in the ingredients.
- **Propyl gallate** (propyl 3,4,5-trihydroxybenzoate). Antioxidant, preservation. Used in oils, meat products, chicken soup base, butter margarine, breakfast cereals, desserts, and chewing gum. In high amounts (2.3% of the diet) short-term studies in rats led to death in 40% of the animals during the first month. Surviving animals showed retarded growth and renal damage at death. May be cancer-causing. Acceptable daily intake set at 0-0.2 milligrams per kilogram body weight.
- **Saccharin** (Sweet 'N Low). Artificial sweetener. Added to beverages (fruit juices and drink mixes). Used as a sugar substitute in individual packets. Processed foods may only have 30 milligrams of saccharin per serving. Causes bladder cancer in rats. There has been some debate about its cancer-causing potential in humans.
- **Salatrim** (Benefat). Fat substitute. Modified fat developed from canola, cottonseed, soybean or sunflower oils by Nabisco. Added to foods as a low-calorie fat substitute. Can be found in reduced fat cookies and chocolate chips. In large amounts (30 grams per day), may cause cramps and nausea.
- **Sodium nitrate, sodium nitrite.** Flavoring agent, food coloring, preservative. Commonly used to preserve color in fish and meats, or keep them pink/red instead of brown. Sodium nitrate has been shown to be toxic in mammals. A single dose

of 1 gram is toxic to humans; eight grams may be fatal and ingestion of 13-15 grams is generally fatal. In the presence of heat and amino acids, as in cooking meat or in the gastro-intestinal tract, these compounds can form cancer-causing agents and these cancer-causing agents have been associated with migraines. Studies demonstrating a link between co-lon cancer and meat consumption may suggest that sodium nitrite is involved. There is also some evidence that eating meats containing nitrites may lead to lung disease (COPD).

- **Sodium silicoaluminate** (sodium aluminosilicate, alumi-num sodium salt, aluminosilicic acid, aluminum sodium silicate). Anti-caking agent. This additive contains both sodium and aluminum. The association of aluminum with Alzheimer's disease remains inconclusive. Avoid aluminum containing additives. Sodium silicate has been shown to pro-duce damage in dog kidneys. Sodium-sensitive individuals should limit intake.

- **Sucralose** (Splenda). Artificial sweetener (I,6-dichloro-I,6-dideosy-B-D-fructofuranosyl-4-chloro-4-deoxy-a-D-galactopyranoside, I',4,6'-trichlorogalactosucrose, trichlorosucrose, and Splenda). Used in several food items. More than 100 studies have been done on sucralose and some of these studies have found that it may trigger mi-graines. It also appears to have adverse side effects on the gut tissue. Sucralose caused DNA damage in the gut of mice and also a reduction of beneficial gut bacteria when given an equivalent acceptable dosage for humans as determined by the US FDA.

- **Sulfites** (potassium bisulfite, potassium metabisulfite, so-dium metabisulfite, sodium sulfite, sulfur dioxide, sodium bisulfite). Antioxidant, antimicrobial dough conditioner, preservative. Highly allergenic ingredient, particularly for those with asthma; can lead to migraines, hives, itching and breathing difficulties. Sulfur dioxide may be especially problematic. Avoid if you are allergic.

- **THBQ** (Tertiary butylhydroquinone, tert-butylhydroquinone). Antioxidant, preservative. Found in a variety of products, including butter, bread, confections, ice cream, margarines, pasta, and sauces. Shown to be cancer-causing in animals.
- **Food Additives You Can Eat**
- Again, the information on additives listed here could change based on new research findings. Please double-check for yourself that this information is still current.
- **Acetic acid.** Acid, flavor enhancer, preservative. Found naturally in plant and animal tissues as a product of carbohydrate fermentation. Safe to consume when diluted and in small amounts such as those found in foods. If ingested in its pure form can cause severe damage (bleeding, ulcers) in the intestines.
- **Agar** (agar-agar). Mucilagenous substance from various seaweed sources. Used extensively in Asian foods and medicinally as a treatment for constipation. May have a laxative effect. Since it swells with water, may promote a feeling of fullness when eaten. May cause an allergic reaction in sensitive people. Avoid if allergic.
- **Alginate** (alginic acid, align, sodium alginate, pacific kelp). Brown seaweed-derived ingredient that can stabilize foam and act as a thickener in products. Sodium alginate is the sodium salt form. Theoretically, due to its ability to trap dietary cholesterol in its gel-like structure, it may have cholesterol-lowering effects. May cause allergic reactions in sensitive individuals. Avoid if allergic.
- **Annatto extract.** Food coloring, flavoring agent. Red food

coloring derived from the tropical achiote tree. Imparts sweet peppery flavor. Has potential to cause allergic reactions in sensitive people. Avoid if allergic.

- **Astaxanthin.** Food coloring, nutrient. Red pigment (carotenoid) found naturally in algae, yeast, and fish (salmon, krill) that can be used to color animal and fish foods. Found in dietary supplements. Potent antioxidant, used throughout the body, especially in the central nervous system. May cause allergic reactions in people who are sensitive to fish or algae. Avoid if allergic.

- **Baking soda.** (bicarbonate of soda, sodium bicarbonate, sodium hydrogen carbonate). Fine white alkaline powder that combines with acidic ingredients or additives (lemon juice, cream of tartar, phosphates) to produce carbon dioxide gas, causing food to rise. Contains sodium. Limit use if you are sodium sensitive.

- **Beeswax.** Honeybees secrete this waxy substance as a part of the honeycomb. Yellow beeswax is made commercially by removing honey from honeycomb, melting the comb, and refining the wax by melting and adding an acid or alkali to remove impurities. Beeswax has a long history of safe use. Some people who may be sensitive to bee-derived products should avoid. Also those who are allergic should avoid.

- **Beet powder.** Food coloring. Dark red powder made from beets.

- **Beta-carotene** (Vitamin A precursor). Antioxidant, food coloring nutrient. Orange pigment (carotenoid) that occurs naturally in fruits and vegetables. High amounts, more likely in supplemental form rather than foods, are not advocated for smokers. Once ingested, it can convert in the body to Vitamin A.

- **Calcium chloride.** Firming agent, flavoring agent. Keeps fruit firm. Found in bottled waters as an electrolyte.

- **Calcium gluconate** (Calcium di-gluconate. Firming agent, nutrient. Contains a small amount of calcium.
- **Calcium or Sodium stearoyl lactylate** (sodium stearoyl fumarate). Slightly sweet white powder made from the combination of lactic acid and the fatty acid, stearic acid, followed by treating it with either calcium hydroxide or sodium hydroxide to make the calcium or sodium salt, respectively. Although rare, lactose-intolerant people may be sensitive to the lactylate. Avoid if lactose-intolerant; sodium-sensitive people should limit the sodium form of this additive.
- **Canthaxanthin.** Antioxidant, food coloring, nutrient. Orange-red pigment (carotenoid) found in crustaceans, fish and eggs. Primarily used as feed additive for animals to produce more intensely colored flesh and egg yolks. May also be found in dietary supplants containing "mixed carotenoids." Levels found added to foods do not seem to result in intake that exceeds the Acceptable Daily Intake (ADI) of up to 0.03 milligrams per kilogram body weight. The amounts found in foods may be too insignificant for health.
- **Carboxymethylcellulose** (Sodium carboxymethylcellulose, cellulose gum, CMC). Odorless, white to yellow, water-soluble plant fiber (cellulose) derivative reacted with an acid. Used as a binder in dietary supplements. Considered a fiber source, used as a laxative in over-the-counter preparations. Sodium-sensitive people should note sodium source coming from sodium carboxymethylcellulose. Sodium-sensitive people should limit or reduce intake of sodium carboxymethylcellulose.
- **Carnauba wax.** Wax obtained from Brazilian carnauba palm. Commercial grades contain saturated fatty acids and alcohols. Acceptable daily intake set at 0-7 milligrams per kilogram body weight.

- **Carrot oil**. Food coloring. Orange, oily extract from carrots. Contains carotenoids like beta-carotene, which may have health promoting effects.
- **Chlorophyll** (CI natural green 3, chlorophyllin). Antioxidant, food coloring. Green pigment found in plants. Chlorophyllin is a stabilized form or chlorophyll made by adding sodium or copper to chlorophyll. Found in dietary supplements. May act as an antioxidant.
- **Phytosterols/phytostanols**. (plantsterols, plantstanols, stanolesters, beta-sitosterol, campesterol, stigmasterol). Nutrient. Cholesterol like compounds found naturally in plant sources like vegetable oils, nuts, vegetables, and seeds. Ester forms are sometimes used in foods since they are more fat soluble. These beneficial additives reduce cholesterol absorption from food and lower LDL (bad) cholesterol in blood by 10-15%. Food products that contain these compounds in certain amounts are allowed to carry an FDA-approved health claim on heart-disease risk.
- **Sodium gluconate**. Sodium salt of gluconic acid produced commercially by glucose fermentation. A fine white crystalline powder added to certain foods, like rice cakes. Contains sodium. If you are sensitive to sodium you should limit your intake of this additive.
- **Sorbic acid**. (calcium sorbate, potassium sorbate, sodium sorbate). Naturally occurring preservative, first identified in unripe berries of Sorbus aucuparia, a plant grown in the northern hemisphere. It prevents mold, yeast and bacterial growth. Sodium, calcium, or potassium salts of sorbic acid are used for their high water solubility. Sorbates are used in a wide array of food and cosmetic products. If you are sensitive to sodium you should limit your intake of this additive.

- **Stevia.** Sweetener. "Stevia" refers to a large plant family, specifically to Stevia rebaudiana Bertoni, also known as sweetleaf. Very sweet. It has been claimed to be 300 times sweeter than sugar. Available in the U.S. as a dietary supplement. There are mixed results on stevia: an older study found that it was weakly mutagenic (caused changes in DNA), while newer studies suggest that it may have healthy benefits like improving blood-sugar response. Recent work indicates it may actually protect DNA and improve immune system functioning. In 2006, the WHO (World Health Organization) concluded that it was not toxic to genes and did not find evidence that it is a caner-causing agent. Used extensively for more than 30 years in countries like Japan and in South America.
- **Succinic acid.** Flavoring agent. Colorless, crystalline acid added to meats and condiments. Found naturally in plant and animal tissues as a part of metabolism.
- **Turmeric** (curcumin). Antioxidant, food coloring. Bright orange-yellow pigment from the root of the plant, Curcuma longa. Contains curcuminoids, which act as antioxidants and may have anti-inflammatory, anti-cancer properties.
- **Vanillin** (methyl vanillin, ethyl vanillin, vanillin acetate). Flavor agent. Vanillin occurs naturally in the vanilla bean, along with hundreds of other compounds. Due to the expense and scarcity of the vanilla bean, vanillin, a synthetic flavoring derived as a waste product of the wood pulp industry, was developed. It is used in in foods and drinks. Sometimes used together with vanilla. This combination extract is found on the food label as "vanilla-vanillin extract." Acceptable daily intake set at 0-10 milligrams per kilogram body weight.
- **Vitamin B1** Nutrient. Water-soluble B vitamin found naturally in yeast, liver, whole grains, vegetables, and meats that

is required in the body to metabolize carbohydrates and for nerve function. Recommended daily allowance (RDA) for adults is 1.2 milligrams for men fourteen years and older and 1.1 milligrams for women eighteen years and older. Ingesting large amounts of coffee and tea can react with thiamin in food, making it inactive. Can be taken in the form of dietary supplement.

- **Vitamin B2** (riboflavin, riboflavin-5-phosphate). Nutrient, colorant, Water-soluble B vitamin that naturally occurs in meat, eggs, vegetables, and milk. Prepared commercially from yeast. Can be synthesized from genetically modified yeast. Found in all living organisms, as it is required for cellular respiration. Indirectly involved in maintaining the integrity of blood cells. RDA for adults is 1.3 milligrams for men 14 years and older and 1.1 milligrams for women 18 years and older. Added to a variety of fortified foods as a nutrient or as a colorant (it has a yellow-orange color). Also found in dietary supplements.
- **Vitamin B3** (niacin, niacinamide, nicotinic acid). Nutrient. Water-soluble B vitamin found in meat, grain beans, vegetables, yeast, milk, and fish. Niacin compounds are used throughout the body to make energy and for more than 200 enzymes involved in energy-transfer reactions. High levels of niacin are available by prescription and as an over-the-counter supplement for high blood fats. RDA for adults is 16 milligrams for men 14 years and older and 14 milligrams for women the same age.
- **Vitamin B6** (pyridoxine, pyridocxine hydrochloride, pyridoxal phosphate, pyridoxal 5 phosphate, pyridoxal-5-phosphate, pyridoxamine, pyridoxine HCI, pyridoxine-5-phosphate). Nutrient. Water-soluble B vitamin found naturally in whole grains, vegetables, nuts, beans, eggs, and meat. In the body,

used for metabolizing fats, proteins, and carbohyudrates. Together with folic acid and vitamin B12, can help reduce blood levels of homocysteine, a compound associated with heart-disease risk. RDA for adults is 1.3 milligrams for women 19-50 years. For men, the RDA is 1.3 milligrams for men 14-50, and 1.7 milligrams for men older than 50.

- **Vitamin C** (ascorbic acid, ascorbate, ascorbyl palmitate, calcium ascorbate, L-ascorbic acid, sodium ascorbate). Acid, antioxidant, nutrient. Water-soluble vitamin naturally occurring in citrus fruits, and can also be chemically synthesized. Biologically necessary for humans for healthy teeth, bones, and blood vessels. Used as an antioxidant. Can inhibit the formation of cancer compounds. RDA for men 19 and older is 95 milligrams, and 75 milligrams for women the same age. Considered to be a safe compound at levels below 2000 mg daily.

- **Vitamin D** (cholecalciferol or vitamin D3; egocalciferol, calciferol or Vitamin D2). Fat-soluble vitamin often referred to as a hormone. Comes in a variety of forms. Food is most commonly supplemented with either ergocalciferol (vitamin D2), from yeast or fungi sources) or cholecalciferol (vitamin D3, from fish-liver oils), which is a more activated form of vitamin D than vitamin D2. Vitamin D can be found in eggs from hens supplemented with vitamin D-containing feed and oily fish. Assists in promoting bone health, together with minerals like calcium. May also play a role in cancer and autoimmune conditions. Likely safe below amounts of 2000 IU daily. Most fortified foods contain 100 IU vitamin D or less.

- **Vitamin E** (d-alpha tocopherol, dl-alpha tocopherol, alpha tocopherol acetate, alpha tocopheryl acetate, d-alpha-tocopheryl acid succinate, d-alpha-tocopheryl succinate, d-alpha tocotrienol, mixed tocopherols, palm tocotrienols, tocopherol, tocopherol acetate, tocopheryl acetate, mixed tocotrienols, vitamin E acetate, vitamin E succinate). Antioxidant, nutrient. A fat-soluble vitamin found naturally in vegetable, oils, fruits, seeds, nuts, grains, eggs, and meat. Wheat germ is a notable source of vitamin E. The "natural" form of vitamin E is designated by the "d" (d-alpha tocopherol) whereas the "synthesized" form is indicated by the "dl" (dl-alpha tocopherol) before the name. The natural form is more available to the body than the synthetic form. Commonly added to fats and oils to prevent rancidity. Many of vitamin E's functions throughout the body may be related to its ability to serve as an antioxidant. Considered to be reasonably safe, depending on the dose added. Levels above 400 IU on a daily basis may require medical supervision.

- **Zeaxanthin.** Food coloring, nutrient. Orange-red powdered pigment found naturally in vegetables, especially corn and leafy greens like kale and collard greens. Accumulates in the retina of the eye. Eating foods high in zeaxanthin may protect against blindness due to degeneration of he part of the retina called the macula. Zeaxanthin often occurs together with another carotenoid, lutein. Acceptable daily intake for either lutein or zeaxanthin separately or collectively is set at 0-2 milligrams per kilogram body weight.

- **Zinc** (zinc chloride, zinc gluconate, zinc methionine sulfate, zinc oxide, zinc stearate, zinc sulfate). Nutrient. Essential element needed for more than 300 enzymes to work in the body, some of them responsible for making DNA. Also important for immune system functioning. High-protein foods like meats, seafood, nuts, legumes, and grains naturally contain zinc. RDA for adults is 11 milligrams for men 14 and older and 8 milligrams for women 19 years and older.

- **Zingerone** (valillylacetone, 4-(4-hydroxy-3-methoxyphenyl) -2-butanone). Flavoring agent. A pungent flavoring agent used to flavor spice oils.

Potential Cancer Causing Food Additives

- Acesulfame-potassium (Sunett®, Sweet One®)
- Artificial coloring
- Aspartame (NutraSweet®, Equal®)
- Butylated Hydroxyanisole (BHA)
- Butylated Hydroxytoluene (BHT)
- Caramel color
- Carrageenan (when degraded in the presence of high heat and fed in large amounts)
- Diacetyl
- Potassium bromate
- Propyl gallate
- Saccharin (Sweet 'N Low®)
- Sodium benzoate (In combination with ascorbic acid, may react under specific conditions to form benzene, a carcinogen)
- Tert-butylhydroquinone (THBQ)

Additives that May Provoke Allergic Reactions

These may cause asthma problems, breathing difficulties, fatigue, headaches, increased hear rate, migraines and skin reactions.

- Agar
- Alginate (alginic acid, algin, sodium alginate, Pacific kelp)
- Annatto extract
- Artificial coloring
- Aspartame (NutraSweet®, Equal®)
- Bromate (calcium bromate, potassium bromate)

- Caffeine
- Calcium propionate
- Carmine
- Cohineal
- Gums (acacia, Arabic, furcellaran, guar, locust bean, tragacanth, xanthan)
- Hydrolyzed vegetable protein (HVP, TVP, hydrolyzed soy protein, hydrolyzed wheat protein, hydrolyzed whey protein, hydrolyzed casein, texturized vegetable protein)
- Inulin
- Isoamyl acetate
- Monosodium glutamate (MSG)
- Neotame
- Quinine
- Sodium benzote (benzoic acid)
- Sodium hexametaphosphate
- Sucralose (Splenda®)
- Sulfites (potassium bisulfate, potassium metabisulfite, sodium metabisulfite, sodium sulfite, sulfur dioxide, sodium bisulfite)

Additives that May Cause Gastrointestinal Effects

These may cause gas, bloating, cramping or changes in bowel movements:

- Agar (agar-agar)
- Alginate (alginic acid, algin, sodium alginate, Pacific kelp)
- Carboxymethylcellulose (socium carboxymethylcellulose)
- Gluten
- Gums (acacia, Arabic, furcellaran, guar, locust bean, tragacanth, xanthan)
- Hydrogenated starch hydrolysate (hydrogenated glucose

syrup, maltitol syrup, sorbitol syrup)
- Inulin
- Sugar alcohols (erythritol, lactitol, maltitol, mannitol, sorbitol, [glucitol], xylitol)
- Olestra (Olean®)
- Polydextrose (Litesse®, Sta-Lite®, Trimcal)
- Salatrim (Benefat®)
- Vitamin C (high amounts have a laxative effect)

Additives Commonly found in "Junk Foods"

- Acesulfame-potassium (Sunett ®, Sweet One®)
- Artificial colorings
- Aspartame (NutraSweet®, Equal®)
- Butylated hydroxyanisole (BHA)
- Butylated hydroxytoluene (BHT)
- Carmel color
- Corn syrup (solids)
- Dextrose
- High-fructose corn syrup (HFCS)
- Invert sugar
- Neotame
- Olestra (Olean®)
- Partially hydrogenated oils (partially hydrogenated vegetable oil, partially hydrogenated soybean oil, partially hydrogenated palm oil)
- Saccharin (Sweet 'N Low®)
- Salatrim (Benefat®)
- Salt (excessive amounts)
- Sodium nitrate
- Sodium nitrite
- Sucralose (Splenda®)

- Sugar (sucrose, cane sugar, brown sugar, raw sugar in excessive amounts)
- Trans Fats

Additives Lactose-Intolerant Individuals Should Avoid:

- All milk-containing products
- Calcium (or Sodium) stearoyl lactylate
- Lactitol
- Lactose

Additives Gluten-Intolerant Individuals Should Avoid:

- Dextrins (wheat-derived: maltodextrin)
- Gluten
- Hydrogenated starch hydrolysate (wheat-derived: hydrogenated glucose syrup, maltitol syrup, sorbitol syrup)
- Hydrolyzed vegetable protein (wheat-derived: HVP, hydrolyzed protein, hydrolyzed wheat protein, TVP, texturized vegetable protein)
- Maltose (barley-derived: dried maltose syrup, maltose syrup, dried malt syrup)
- Modified food starch (wheat-derived)
- Monon- and Di-glycerides (wheat carrier)

Additives Sodium-Sensitive Individuals Should Limit

- All additives with "sodium" in the name
- All additives with "salt" in the name
- Aluminosilicic acid (aluminum sodium salt, aluminum sodium silicate, disodium citrate)
- Baking soda (bicarbonate of soda, sodium hydrogen carbonate, sodium bicarbonate)

Chapter 2
Clean Eating Grocery List

Fruit
Any fruit in season
Apples
Avocado
Banana
Blackberries
Blueberries
Cherries
Grapefruit
Grapes
Kiwi
Lemons
Limes
Mango
Nectarines
Papaya
Peach
Pears
Pineapple
Plums
Pomegranates
Raspberries
Strawberries
Watermelon

Grains/Beans
Black beans (not canned)
Black bean spaghetti
Brown rice

Brown rice spaghetti
Buckwheat
Cannelini beans (not canned)
Chickpeas
Garbanzo beans
Kidney beans
Lentils
Lima beans (not canned)
Millet
Navy beans (not canned)
Steel-cut oats
Peas
Pinto beans (not canned)
Quinoa
Tahini
Tempeh

Sweeteners
Blackstrap molasses
Local raw honey
Pure maple syrup
Raw dark agave nectar

Meat/Poultry
Albacore tuna (in water)
Beef, grass fed
Bison
Chicken breast
Cod

Eggs
Halibut
Lean ground turkey
Lean ground chicken
Nitrate free bacon (watch the sodium contents)
Salmon, Alaskan
Sardines

Nuts/Seeds
Almonds
Cashews
Chia seeds
Flaxseed
Natural almond butter
Natural peanut butter
Pine nuts
Sunflower seeds
Pecans (raw, no salt)
Pistachios (raw, no salt)
Pumpkin seeds (raw, no salt)
Sesame seeds (raw, no salt)
Sunflower seeds (raw, no salt)
Walnuts (raw, no salt)

Condiments/Oils
Apple cider vinegar
Black pepper
Coconut oil
Extra virgin olive oil
Flaxseed oil
Sesame oil

Liquids
Fruit infused water
Green tea
Herbal tea
Unsweetened coconut milk
Unsweetened almond milk
Water

Herbs - Fresh
Any herbs and spices (not table salt)
Basil
Cayenne/Chili pepper
Cilantro/parsley
Cinnamon
Cumin
Dill
Ginger
Mint
Mustard seeds
Oregano
Pink Himalayan salt
Red pepper flakes
Rosemary
Thyme
Turmeric

Vegetables
Any vegetable in season
Alfalfa sprouts
Asparagus
Beets

Bok Choy
Broccoli
Brussels sprouts
Cabbage
Carrots

Collard greens
Green beans
Kale
Spinach
Zucchini

How to Take your Measurements

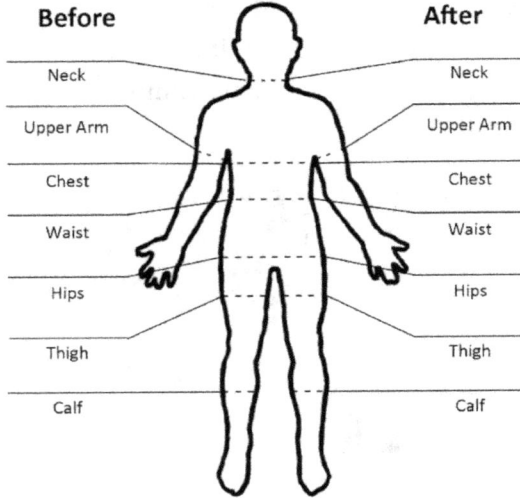

Before   **After**

Before	After
Neck	Neck
Upper Arm	Upper Arm
Chest	Chest
Waist	Waist
Hips	Hips
Thigh	Thigh
Calf	Calf

Measurement Tracking Sheet

Year:	Date:	Date:	Date:	Date:	Date:	Date:
Neck						
Biceps (left)						
Biceps (right)						
Chest						
Waist						
Hips						
Thigh (left)						
Thigh (right)						
Calf (left)						
Calf (right)						
Weight						

Bibliography

Tip for the day; Cleaning Fruit – Chemical – free and easy. (20123, May 17). Retrieved from Daily Inspirations for Healthy Living: http://suhanijain.com/2013/05/17/tip-for-the-daycleaning-fruit-chemical-free-and-easy/

Are abs REALLY made in the kitchen? (2013, July 11). Retrieved from myfitnesspal: http://www.myfitnesspal.com/topics/show/1042031-are-abs-really-made-in-the-kitchen

All 48 fruits and vegetables with pesticide residue data. (2014, April). Retrieved from Environmental Working Group: http://www.ewg.org/foodnews/list.php

Bod Pod. (2014, July 9). Retrieved from HearthStone Health + Fitness: http://www.hearthstonehealthandfitness.com/bod-pod.html

Detox 101. (2014, June 25). Retrieved from Ultimate health Trends: http://body.ultimatehealthtrends.com/detox-101/

Food additives. (2014, May 19). Retrieved from University of Maryland Medical Center: http://umm.edu/health/medical/ency/articles/food-additives

Reading Food Nutrition Labels. (2014, June 12). Retrieved from American Heart Association: http://www.heart.org/HEARTORG/GettingHealthy/NutritionCenter/HeartSmartShopping/Reading-Food-Nutrition-Labels_UCM_300132_Article.jsp

Start Your Own Walking Group. (2014, April 3). Retrieved from Every Body Walk!: http://everybodywalk.org/start-your-own-walking-group

The Difference Between USDA Organic and Non-GMO Verified Seal. (2014, June 8). Retrieved from Boston Organics: http://bostonorganics.com/wordpress/2013/10/24/avoid-gmos-the-difference-between-organic-and-non-gmo-labels/

Time Your Carbs Right. (2014, August). *Oxygen*, p. 34.

Types of Carbohydrates. (2014, July 5). Retrieved from SuperSkinnyMe: http://www.superskinnyme.com/types-of-carbohydrates.html

Amy. (2013, February 5). *30 Bananas A Day*. Retrieved from Food Combininig: http://www.30bananasaday.com/photo/food-combining?xg_source=activity

Beth. (2013, March 18). *10 Benefits to Drinking Warm Lemon Water Every Morning*. Retrieved from Tasty Yummies: http://tasty-yummies.com/2013/03/18/10-benefits-to-drinking-warm-lemon-water-every-morning/

Breene, S. (2013, March 27). *13 Mental Health Benefits Of Exercise* . Retrieved from Huff Post: http://www.huffingtonpost.com/2013/03/27/mental-health-benefits-exercise_n_2956099.html

Bruso, J. (2014, February 7). *List of Complex Carbs vs. Simple Carbs*. Retrieved from Livestrong.com: http://www.livestrong.com/article/291272-list-of-complex-carbs-vs-simple-carbs/

Christyn. (2012). *Abs Are Made In The Kitchen!* Retrieved from thefitnessfashionista: http://www.thefitnessfashionista.com/abs-are-made-in-the-kitchen

Clean Eating. (n.d.). Retrieved April 14, 2014, from Clean

Eating: http://www.cleaneatingmag.com/food-health/
food-and-health-news/what-is-clean-eating/

Frank-Tuomey, R. (2012, July 3). *The Essential Grocery List for 'Clean' Eating*. Retrieved from Mind Body Green: http://www.mindbodygreen.com/0-5353/The-Essential-Grocery-List-for-Clean-Eating.html

Fullen, B. (2013, April 10). *Homemade Vegetable and Fruit Soak*. Retrieved from Live Healthier: http://barbfullen.wordpress.com/2013/04/10/homemade-vegetable-and-fruit-soak/

Grand, T. (2013, September 30). *10 Questions People Ask Personal Trainers*. Retrieved from fitknitchick: http://fitknitchick.com/2013/09/30/10-questions-people-ask-personal-trainers/

Hanly, L. (2013, October 21). *How Long Does it Take to Change Your Body After Working Out?* Retrieved from Livingstrong.com: http://www.livestrong.com/article/438047-how-long-does-it-take-to-change-your-body-after-working-out/

Jampolis, D. M. (2011, September 30). *Expert Q&Q*. Retrieved from CNN Health: http://www.cnn.com/2011/HEALTH/expert.q.a/09/30/body.fat.testing.jampolis/

Jaret, P. (2014, June 25). *Reading the Ingredient Label: What to Look For*. Retrieved from WebMD: http://www.webmd.com/food-recipes/features/healthy-ingredients

Lyman, A. (2014, June 2). *What Is a Gait Analysis?* Retrieved from Active: http://www.active.com/running/articles/what-is-a-gait-analysis

Merriam-Webster. (n.d.). Retrieved May 19, 2014, from Merriam-Webster: http://www.merriam-webster.com/

Minich, Ph.D., C.N., D. M. (2009). *An A-Z Guide ot Food Additives*. San Francisco: Conari Press.

BIBLIOGRAPHY

NON GMO PROJECT. (n.d.). Retrieved April 24, 2014, from
NON GMO PROJECT: http://www.nongmoproject.org/
learn-more/what-is-gmo/

Staff, M. C. (2014, February 5). *Exercise: 7 benefits of regular physical
activity.* Retrieved from Mayo Clinic: http://www.mayoclinic.
org/healthy-living/fitness/in-depth/exercise/art-20048389

Styles, S. (2014, June 25). *Healthy Eating.* Retrieved from SFGate:
http://healthyeating.sfgate.com/clean-fruits-vegetables-vine-
gar-8777.html

United States Deparment of Agriculture. (n.d.). Retrieved April 24,
2014, from Agricultureal Marketing Service: http://www.ams.
usda.gov/AMSv1.0/NOPOrganicStandards

USDA United States Department of Agriculture. (n.d.). Retrieved
April 24, 2014, from USDA United States Department of
Agriculture: http://www.usda.gov/wps/portal/usda/usdahome?c
ontentidonly=true&contentid=organic-agriculture.html

Walters, J. (2014, June 30). *What You Forgot to Ask Your Personal
Trainer.* Retrieved from SPARKPEOPLE: http://www.spark-
people.com/resource/fitness_articles.asp?id=1369

Amy. (2013, February 5). *30 Bananas A Day.* Retrieved from
Food Combininig: http://www.30bananasaday.com/photo/
food-combining?xg_source=activity

Are abs REALLY made in the kitchen? (2013, July 11). Retrieved
from myfitnesspal: http://www.myfitnesspal.com/topics/
show/1042031-are-abs-really-made-in-the-kitchen

Beth. (2013, March 18). *10 Benefits to Drinking Warm Lemon Water
Every Morning.* Retrieved from Tasty Yummies: http://tasty-
yummies.com/2013/03/18/10-benefits-to-drinking-warm-
lemon-water-every-morning/

Bruso, J. (2014, February 7). *List of Complex Carbs vs. Simple Carbs.* Retrieved from Livestrong.com: http://www.livestrong.com/article/291272-list-of-complex-carbs-vs-simple-carbs/

Christyn. (2012). *Abs Are Made In The Kitchen!* Retrieved from thefitnessfashionista: http://www.thefitnessfashionista.com/abs-are-made-in-the-kitchen

Detox 101. (2014, June 25). Retrieved from Ultimate health Trends: http://body.ultimatehealthtrends.com/detox-101/

Frank-Tuomey, R. (2012, July 3). *The Essential Grocery List for 'Clean' Eating.* Retrieved from Mind Body Green: http://www.mindbodygreen.com/0-5353/The-Essential-Grocery-List-for-Clean-Eating.html

Time Your Carbs Right. (2014, August). *Oxygen*, p. 34.

Types of Carbohydrates. (2014, July 5). Retrieved from SuperSkinnyMe: http://www.superskinnyme.com/types-of-carbohydrates.html

BOD POD®. (2014, July 9). Retrieved from HearthStone Health + Fitness: http://www.hearthstonehealthandfitness.com/bod-pod.html

Breene, S. (2013, March 27). *13 Mental Health Benefits Of Exercise* . Retrieved from Huff Post: http://www.huffingtonpost.com/2013/03/27/mental-health-benefits-exercise_n_2956099.html

Grand, T. (2013, September 30). *10 Questions People Ask Personal Trainers.* Retrieved from fitknitchick: http://fitknitchick.com/2013/09/30/10-questions-people-ask-personal-trainers/

Hanly, L. (2013, October 21). *How Long Does it Take to Change Your Body After Working Out?* Retrieved from Livingstrong.com: http://www.livestrong.com/

article/438047-how-long-does-it-take-to-change-your-body-after-working-out/

Jampolis, D. M. (2011, September 30). *Expert Q&Q*. Retrieved from CNN Health: http://www.cnn.com/2011/HEALTH/expert.q.a/09/30/body.fat.testing.jampolis/

Lyman, A. (2014, June 2). *What Is a Gait Analysis?* Retrieved from Active: http://www.active.com/running/articles/what-is-a-gait-analysis

Mayo Clinic Staff (2014, February 5). *Exercise: 7 benefits of regular physical activity*. Retrieved from Mayo Clinic: http://www.mayoclinic.org/healthy-living/fitness/in-depth/exercise/art-20048389

Start Your Own Walking Group. (2014, April 3). Retrieved from Every Body Walk!: http://everybodywalk.org/start-your-own-walking-group

Walters, J. (2014, June 30). *What You Forgot to Ask Your Personal Trainer*. Retrieved from SPARKPEOPLE: http://www.sparkpeople.com/resource/fitness_articles.asp?id=1369

http://www.mindbodygreen.com/0-14685/spiced-summer-vegetable-casserole.html

http://shrinkingkitchen.com/homemade-low-sodium-taco-seasoning/

http://www.mindbodygreen.com/0-14564/homemade-pineapple-juice-with-a-cinnamon-twist.html

http://www.thegraciouspantry.com/clean-eating-chicken-cucumber-toss/#ixzz38Cyudtf3

http://www.thegraciouspantry.com/clean-eating-italian-dressing/#ixzz38CyLmL5C

http://www.muscle-fitness.co.uk/nutrition/

article/6-healthy-breakfast-alternatives

http://www.sportsrecipes.com/

http://www.oxygenmag.com/almond-oat-granola-bars/

http://ifoodreal.com/tex-mex-spaghetti-squash-boats-recipe/

http://www.muscleandfitnesshers.com/recipes/salad-days?page=3.

http://www.health.com/health/recipe/0,,10000000635576,00.html

http://www.health.com/health/recipe/0,,10000000521997,00.html

http://www.themotherhuddle.com/
classic-guacamole-plus-a-great-tip-for-preparing-it/

http://www.food.com/recipe/
turkey-breakfast-sausage-patties-100408

http://www.seriouseats.com/recipes/2011/03/grilling-smashed-po-
tatoes.html

http://www.oxygenmag.com/slideshow/9-meals-for-your-abs/9/

http://www.coquettishmish.com/2012/10/healthy-naturally-fla-
vored-water.html

Ruel, D., & Losie, K. (2013). *Metabolic Cooking.* Retrieved from
Metabolic Cooking: http://www.MetabolicCooking.com

www.ingramcontent.com/pod-product-compliance
Lightning Source LLC
Chambersburg PA
CBHW061009280326
41935CB00009B/888